Dumping Iron

How to Ditch This Secret Killer and Reclaim Your Health

by

P. D. Mangan

Phalanx Press

Disclaimer: This book contains general information about medical conditions and treatments. The information is not advice, and should not be treated as such. The medical information in this book is provided "as is" without any representations or warranties, express or implied. The author makes no representations or warranties in relation to the medical information in this book. The author does not warrant that the medical information in this book is complete, true, accurate, up-to-date, or non-misleading. You must not rely on the information in this book as an alternative to medical advice from your doctor or other professional healthcare provider.

If you have any specific questions about any medical matter you should consult your doctor or other professional healthcare provider. If you think you may be suffering from any medical condition, you should seek immediate medical attention. You should never delay seeking medical advice, disregard medical advice, or discontinue medical treatment because of information in this book.

Copyright 2016 by P. D. Mangan

Table of Contents

What the Experts Say About *Dumping Iron*	4
Foreword	7
Preface: Confronting Ferrotoxic Disease	9
Author's Preface	14
Introduction: Iron, the Secret Killer	17
1: Iron Causes Aging	23
2: Iron and Heart Disease	41
3: Iron Causes Cancer	49
4: Iron Is Linked to Brain Diseases and Cognitive Decline	60
5: Diabetes, Obesity, and Iron	70
6: Iron is implicated in many other diseases	79
7: How to take control of your iron and your health	103
8: Conclusion	146
Appendix: The Men Who Discovered the Iron Connection	150
Acknowledgments	155
About the Author	156
Bibliography	159

What the Experts Say About *Dumping Iron*

"*Dumping Iron* by P. D. Mangan is a must read by anybody interested in maintaining optimal health, including those in the medical field. Iron overload is an exceedingly common malady in the population and it is easily diagnosed, but it is under-addressed. It leads to heart disease, diabetes, cancer and numerous other chronic and debilitating illnesses. The good news is that iron excess can be prevented and readily treated, which results in a decreased risk of many diseases and improvement in overall health and vitality. *Dumping Iron* clearly tells us how to achieve these goals."

— Luca Mascitelli, M.D., Lieutenant Colonel, Italian Army, and author of numerous scientific papers on iron and health.

"In *Dumping Iron*, Dennis Mangan has provided the reader access to a massive scientific data pool linking body iron overload to major diseases of mankind... I submit that *Dumping Iron* should be required reading in science and nutrition for high school and above. The ultimate triumph of *Dumping Iron* might be an informed public that will increasingly access ferritin test screening, and health care providers better prepared to interpret tests of iron status, particularly the ferritin level. Acknowledgment of risks of iron overload and proper product labeling might lead to reduced public iron intoxication and improved population health to a degree that would be no less than monumental!"

— Leo Zacharski, M.D., Professor of Medicine, Geisel School of Medicine, Dartmouth College

Dennis Mangan's revolutionary new book Dumping Iron: How to Ditch This Secret Killer and Reclaim Your Health is a must read even for the most informed Health and Fitness professional.

For those of us writing in the medical/anti-aging field, it is imperative to cite your work, as much of the research is newly available and stands directly in the face of 'modern medical advice'. Dennis's work is authoritative and his writing style is clear and thought provoking. In fact, I don't believe there has been a written book on the risks of elevated iron levels so extensively researched- offering the reader more than 120 citations.

His thesis that excess iron accumulates in the blood as one ages leading to cellular and biological inflammation and ultimately the diseases of aging (heart disease, cancer, and cognitive decline), is impossible to dispute. So much so, I'm going to share it with my inner circle and implore them to get their ferritin levels tested.

Do yourself a favor and read this book immediately. The overall success of your aging process and the extension of your life may depend on it.

— Jay Campbell, author of The Definitive Testosterone Replacement Therapy MANual

Foreword

By E. D. Weinberg, PhD

Iron has been compared to fire. A small amount of fire is quite useful in our stoves and furnaces. But when fire is ravaging the contents and walls of our homes... BEWARE. In this informative book, Dennis Mangan makes clear the devastation that can be caused by excessive/misplaced iron in the tissues and walls of our bodies. We learn that for essentially all diseases – infections, cancers, Alzheimer's, Parkinson's, diabetes, gout, osteoporosis, cardiovascular ills, and more – that the iron burden is a dangerous risk factor.

But equally important, the author describes a variety of well tested methods that are readily available to neutralize the iron peril. Adoption of even a few of these methods can remarkably decrease iron-catalyzed disease episodes, enhance well-being, and, not least, increase longevity.

During the past sixty years, the many hundreds of published studies of iron toxicity have consistently demonstrated the hazard of ignoring the dangerous metal. An early report summarized it well: "The iron heart is not a strong heart; it is a very weak one."[1]

E.D. Weinberg is Professor Emeritus of Biology at Indiana University, and the author of over 140 scientific papers, many of them on the role of iron in disease.

---

[1] Biya LM & Roberts WC "Iron in the heart" Am J Med (1971) 51:202-221

Preface: Confronting Ferrotoxic Disease

By Leo Zacharski, M.D.

In "Dumping Iron", Dennis Mangan has provided the reader access to a massive scientific data pool linking body iron overload to major diseases of mankind.

Iron, in excess of requirements for normal respiration, generates highly toxic hydroxyl radicals contributory to "inflammation and oxidative stress responsible for the grand global health challenges: diabetes, cancer, neurodegenerative disorders, hypertension and cardiovascular disease."[1] The very thought that so pedestrian and easily controlled a culprit might be linked to premature suffering and death may explain partly why the concept of "ferrotoxic disease" has been embraced reluctantly or not at all.[2] Among well-documented health hazards, iron excess must remain one of the world's best kept secrets.

Using masterful prose, Mangan has outlined the magnitude of the problem and described factors responsible for "iron blindness" among health care providers and within the general public. This volume can claim status as an iron nutrition owner's manual.

The degree to which iron is noxious is determined by the dose times the duration: the more iron on-board and the longer it remains, the greater the risk. "Normal" iron levels represented by ferritin are those levels associated with minimum disease risk and maximum longevity.

> The very thought that so pedestrian and easily controlled a culprit might be linked to premature suffering and death may explain partly why the concept of "ferrotoxic disease" has been embraced reluctantly or not at all.

Several epidemiological studies have shown increased longevity associated with ferritin below an upper threshold of about 80 to 90 ng/ml, the plateau in post-menopausal women (shown in the first figure in this book) that is also conducive to older age in men – those with higher levels have dropped out of the population by dying. Plots of paired values for the ferritin and hemoglobin obtained from a large clinical trial of iron reduction showed that rising ferritin levels up to about 80 ng/ml are associated with rising hemoglobin levels within the normal range, indicating use of iron for red cell oxygen transport. Above the 80 ng/ml cut-off, ferritin levels continue to rise but without physiologic correspondence.

Ferritin levels are a continuum and susceptibility to iron toxicity thus may commence at ferritin levels mistakenly considered to be within the "reference range" used commonly. This explains why much higher ferritin levels are more clearly disease-associated while levels in the 100 to 150 ng/ml range "mysteriously" appear in some, but not all, studies as disease-associated.[3]

The tragedy of ferrotoxic disease is compounded by unnecessary ingestion of highly absorbable iron supplements by an unwary public, for a disease that most people do not have (iron deficiency), and without their knowledge or consent. Recommendations for "minimum daily requirements" for iron used to justify supplementation are based on estimates applied blindly to a population without consideration of existing body iron levels.[4] Iron supplementation has also been justified based on the existence of "small pale red cells" in populations only a small fraction of which have iron deficiency. Thus, Blacks may appear to have iron deficiency based on red cell morphology but they do not; they have genetically-determined variant red cell hemoglobinization and iron excess.[5] Oriental populations commonly have thalassemia or hemoglobin E resulting in similar red cell morphology, but also have iron excess rather than deficiency. Supplement use in such populations has no effect on hemoglobin levels but rather drives up ferritin levels increasing risk of ferrotoxicity.[6]

Note in the first graph in this book that low risk ferritin levels in young adult males and pre-menopausal females rise into the at-risk range in middle-aged males and post-menopausal females. The imperceptibly slow rise in ferritin levels of about 3 to 5 ng/ml per year could easily be accounted for by ubiquitous but inappropriate iron supplementation of processed foods.[7] This increase need not occur.

Pharmaceutical companies have no incentive to test treatment hypotheses with no prospect of payback. Federal funding agencies have shown little interest in studying the therapeutic/preventive value of shifting potentially noxious excess iron out of storage sites into a physiologic (red cell) compartment, as is achieved with phlebotomy. Potent pharmaceutical iron binding drugs (chelators) do not distinguish between physiological and non-physiological (excessive) iron, and their use may be accompanied by significant toxicity.

I submit that "Dumping Iron" should be required reading in science and nutrition for high school and above. The ultimate triumph of "Dumping Iron" might be an informed public that will increasingly access ferritin test screening, and health care providers better prepared to interpret tests of iron status, particularly the ferritin level. Acknowledgment of risks of iron overload and proper product labeling might lead to reduced public iron intoxication and improved population health to a degree that would be no less than monumental!

Dr. Leo Zacharski is Professor of Medicine, Geisel School of Medicine at Dartmouth College, and manages an iron overload clinic at the Hitchcock Hospital, Lebanon, NH.

Author's Preface

Even though I only started researching the topic of iron and health within the past year, I no longer remember how I stumbled upon it.

I recall that many years ago I read about how the late Dr. Jerome Sullivan, a pathologist, first theorized that men had higher rates of heart disease than women because they have more iron in their bodies. It was a fascinating theory, and so much more compelling, I thought, than the cholesterol hypothesis.

I've long been skeptical of much of mainstream health conventional wisdom; for example, the cholesterol hypothesis of heart disease; the claim that running and jogging are the best forms of exercise; the idea that saturated fat harms our health; and that eating too much is the cause of obesity ("calories in, calories out").

But the idea that too much iron harms us is in a different league. It's something almost no one knows about.

Suppose you're a health conscious person, and you exercise

regularly, you make sure you don't become overweight, you avoid junk food, get eight hours of sleep a night, get regular checkups. You take vitamin D and magnesium, maybe even fish oil.

But you've missed something, because you don't know about it. That's because hardly anyone, even the most health conscious, knows or discusses it.

That missing element is iron. No matter how much you exercise, watch what you eat, and so on, if you don't prevent your iron from becoming too high, you're missing a major element of health that could make all the difference.

Controlling your iron means controlling your risk of a heart attack, cancer, diabetes, Parkinson's and Alzheimer's diseases, infections, even wrinkled skin and gout.

The information and scientific studies supporting the claim that excess iron damages health are out there, but you need to look for them. It's hardly discussed at all in mainstream health writing. Most likely, even your doctor doesn't know or care. He or she will be prescribing you a statin or putting you on other potentially damaging, expensive drugs, and all the while a high iron level could be the real problem, and slowly killing you.

Since there's next to no money to be made from dealing with excess iron, pharmaceutical companies are unlikely to pursue this line of research, and for the same reason most people are unlikely to hear about it.

The experience of researching iron and health can be surreal. You discover how important it is, yet hardly anyone, even the most educated health professional, knows it.

I've heard from people who have very high iron levels, over 1000 – I'll explain exactly what that means later – and whose doctors hardly cared. The doctor of a friend of mine assured her that there was no health benefit to lowering iron through blood donation, which is patently false. If you are neither iron deficient nor grossly and obviously iron overloaded, then doctors don't care. Yet iron can cause illness when neither of these conditions are in place.

In this book, I've documented the information I've presented and the claims that I've made. While scientific citations may be an annoyance to some readers, they're especially necessary in this case. If someone (me) is telling them something radical, such as the iron which no one else says is a problem is killing them, then that someone better be able to back up his statements.

My aim with this book is to spread knowledge of the connection between iron and health, and hopefully to bring better health to millions of people.

I can honestly say that this could be one of the most important health books that you'll ever read.

Introduction: Iron, the Secret Killer

Iron in our food and in our bodies is a secret killer and may be among the greatest causes of ill health.

It's a secret because

- hardly anyone knows what their iron levels are, a critically important piece of information

- there are no symptoms from excess iron alone; the only symptoms are from the disease, such as cancer or a heart attack, that iron causes

- the fact that excess iron causes disease, aging, and cognitive decline – the breakdown of the brain – is known to very few, including most doctors.

Iron is a required nutrient

All forms of life, humans included, require nutrients from their food and their environments in order to live, to grow, and to reproduce. Without them, illness or death result. We need protein, certain fats, vitamins, and minerals, because we can't make them ourselves.

Among the minerals, we need iron – the same iron that's used to make steel.

All living things use iron as a critical element in biological systems. Its ability to readily react with other elements, the same chemical reaction involved in rust, means that living organisms can use it for important functions such as carrying oxygen in the blood and in energy production.

When humans don't get enough iron from their food, they can become ill, a prominent illness being iron-deficiency anemia. In this disorder, a lack of iron means that the body cannot make enough hemoglobin, the crucial component of red blood cells that carries oxygen. Iron-deficiency anemia can cause fatigue, shortness of breath, and in children, can stunt growth and development. In a natural environment, the environment that humans evolved in, dietary iron was a scarce resource, and that scarcity as well as the grave consequences of iron deficiency means that we have evolved to grab and hold on to iron. When we eat food that contains iron, we absorb it into the body where it's used for vital biological processes. Then, in most cases, we never let go of it.

Evolution and iron

New evidence is coming to light that women with higher

body iron stores have higher fertility – they have more children. As a consequence, natural selection would favor those genes that caused higher iron status in women. Humans are inclined to seek out sources of iron; for instance, high-iron foods may taste better. (Think of the difference in taste between beef and chicken.) However, the level of iron that promotes female fertility is much lower than the iron-overload levels we discuss in this book; only minimal levels are necessary for fertility, levels that in the modern West we easily attain.

Formerly, there were few adverse consequences to our physiological avidity for iron and our inability to get rid of it. Women lost blood through the menstrual cycle and childbirth, wounds and intestinal parasites also caused blood loss, and perhaps most importantly, most people did not live past middle age, when the consequences of excess iron accumulation become evident. Natural selection – evolution – never had reason to penalize us for excess iron. It just didn't care if we lived past the age when we had our children. Now that we do, excess iron is a problem.

Iron accumulates as we age

Humans have no controlled way of getting rid of iron from their bodies. If we have an excessive amount, certain hormones cause a decrease in the absorption of iron from food, but the body cannot actively remove it.

The result is that as we get older, iron accumulates in our bodies, often to levels that damage health.

In the developed world, humans no longer live in an environment in which iron is scarce. In fact, iron is difficult to avoid, since in many countries – like the U.S. – iron is required by law to be added to food such as flour, corn meal, and rice.

Our biology, evolved in an iron-scarce environment, can now work against us in our new, iron-rich environment.

The chemical quality that makes iron essential for living things, its ease of reaction, also makes it dangerous. Iron is a potent pro-oxidant, and can react with biological structures, such as proteins and cell membranes, and damage them. Damage accumulates, causing aging and disease.

When accumulated in excess, as it is in many, maybe even the majority, of people in the Western world, iron may be one of the most important causes of aging and disease.

If iron is a major cause of aging and disease, why don't we hear more about it? Much of the research on iron and disease is relatively recent, so this partly explains why this isn't more widely known. Doctors and scientists also have favored other theories of disease, such as cholesterol being the cause of heart disease, and they won't easily give up on these theories. As the physicist Max Planck said, "Science advances one funeral at a time."

Another reason for the lack of diffusion of this knowledge as it concerns aging is that many people, including many scientists and other educated people, think of aging as just something that happens and that little can be done about.

Our culture has promoted iron as a source of strength and vitality, and this may be another reason for the under-recognition of iron in aging and disease. Many people pop iron supplements in the belief that it's good for them. Doctors sometimes prescribe it for no very good reason. Little consideration has been given to the dangers of excess iron.

A list of conditions and diseases that iron causes or exacerbates includes:

- cancer
- heart disease
- type 1, type 2, and gestational diabetes, and the metabolic syndrome
- obesity
- hypertension
- aging
- sarcopenia (muscle wasting)
- osteoporosis
- Alzheimer's disease

- Parkinson's disease
- liver disease
- kidney disease
- infections
- macular degeneration (a cause of blindness)
- gout

This book will show that excess iron is a major cause of aging and disease, and that many or even most adults have far too much iron in their bodies. This information will be presented as non-technically as possible, but scientific citations are provided.

I'll also tell you what you can do about excess iron: how to avoid it, and how to get rid of it if you have it.

This book could save you from much pain and suffering from diseases that are caused by too much iron. It could also help you slow the aging process, so that you can live many more years, free of illness, than you would otherwise.

1: Iron Causes Aging

Aging is a process which causes our bodies to accumulate damage beyond our natural ability to repair it. When our bodies are damaged, they don't function as well, and so aging means an increase in, or a greater tendency to, illness and disease.

Outside of the infectious diseases of childhood, older people have much greater rates of almost every illness than do younger people.

But what causes aging? Scientists have formulated many theories as to how our bodies lose the ability to repair themselves and allow damage to build up. Rather than list all of them, let's look at calorie restriction, since this intervention provides important clues as to how aging works.

Calorie restriction decreases iron and slows aging

Calorie restriction is the most potent, robust intervention for extending the lifespan of laboratory animals; calorie restriction retards aging. By discovering how calorie restriction works, we can gain insight into the aging process.

In calorie restriction, animals are fed from 10% to 50% fewer calories than they would normally eat, or would like to eat, and they live up to 50% longer than normally fed animals. This phenomenon has been tested and proven in a wide range of animals, from microscopic worms (*C. elegans*), to rodents, to monkeys.

Human data using calorie restriction is somewhat lacking, since humans live much longer than most lab animals, and not many people have been restricting their food long enough to see results; but so far, several studies indicate that people who restrict their food intake have much better health. They have better insulin sensitivity, lower amounts of body fat, good heart health, and so on.

Much research on calorie restriction has focused on its effect on growth hormone, which it decreases. In addition, calorie restriction decreases inflammation and oxidative damage, improves cell function, and increases autophagy (the cellular self-cleaning and recycling process). All of these processes are strongly associated with aging, so controlling them slows aging.

Calorie restriction also results in a much lower level of iron in aged animals. This may be one of the most important ways that it slows aging.

Lab rats that are food restricted by 40% accumulate far

lower levels of iron in their bodies as they age.[8] The rats also have much lower levels of aging damage.

This is important because it shows that:

1. calorie restriction slows aging;
2. calorie restriction impedes iron accumulation in animals;
3. less iron in the food-restricted animals resulted in much less damage.

Therefore, iron promotes aging, and restricting iron impedes it.

Yeast are microorganisms that scientists have often used in aging studies. They resemble mammalian cells in many important ways, they can be calorie-restricted, and they live much longer when they are.

Yeast that are calorie-restricted accumulate virtually no more iron when they age than they have when young. Yeast that are fully fed accumulate four to five times as much iron, and develop high levels of oxidative damage to important cellular structures, such as proteins.[9] The accumulation of iron ages and kills them.

As they age, humans, especially men, can also easily accumulate four to five times as much iron as when young.

Some scientists believe that the decreased intake of a single amino acid, methionine, accounts for much or all of the effects of calorie restriction. When animals are restricted in methionine, without being otherwise food-restricted, they live longer. But when scientists *add* methionine to the diet of a lab animal, they accumulate much more iron in their bodies. The evidence from methionine and lifespan points to iron as a causative factor of aging.[10]

The next test would be to see whether preventing animals from accumulating iron, without restricting their food, extends their lifespan. When tea leaves, which strongly inhibit the absorption of iron from food, were added to the food of fruit flies, they lived more than 20% longer, while eating all the food they wanted.[11]

When researchers induce "iron starvation" in the worm *C. elegans*, it lives longer, and when they supplement their food with iron, it ages faster and dies younger.[12]

So, we know that less iron means less damage, and less aging.

Polyphenols, which are plant compounds that are known to have beneficial health effects, provide further evidence that iron accelerates aging and disease. Some of the more well-known polyphenols are EGCG (from green tea), quercetin (found in onions), and curcumin (from the spice turmeric). These (and others) have been termed "calorie-restriction mimetics", since they affect many of the same biological processes as calorie restriction.

All of these chelate (pronounced "key-late") iron, which

means that they bind to it and remove it from cells, and the two, chelator and iron, are then excreted.[13] It is no coincidence that they both remove iron and improve health, and in some cases promote longer life; the removal of iron is intrinsic to their health benefits.

Iron and the Blue Zones

The so-called Blue Zones are places where the populations have high numbers of very old people. Scientists have studied their diets, physical activity, family and social ties, and other factors to try to understand why more people in the Blue Zones live longer.

One study looked at the iron levels in very old and middle-aged people in one of the Blue Zones, the Mediterranean island Sardinia. The very old people, which included nonagenarians and centenarians, had substantially less iron, about 40% less, in their blood than the middle-aged, which suggests that one of the reasons people live that long is due to less iron. Those with higher iron presumably have a higher death rate, and fewer of them live into very old age. In fact, of the seven different metals measured, the two with the highest inverse relationship with age were iron and selenium.[14]

Whatever environmental or genetic factors that lead to longer life among the very old of Sardinia also causes them to accumulate less iron as they age, and this could be precisely why they live so long.

Why women live longer than men

In general, iron harms men more than it harms women.

Women live an average of four years longer than men in the U.S., although that has narrowed from six years longer just a few decades ago. Women also live longer than men in most of the world.

Why is that? A plausible case can be made that the difference is due to lower iron levels in women.

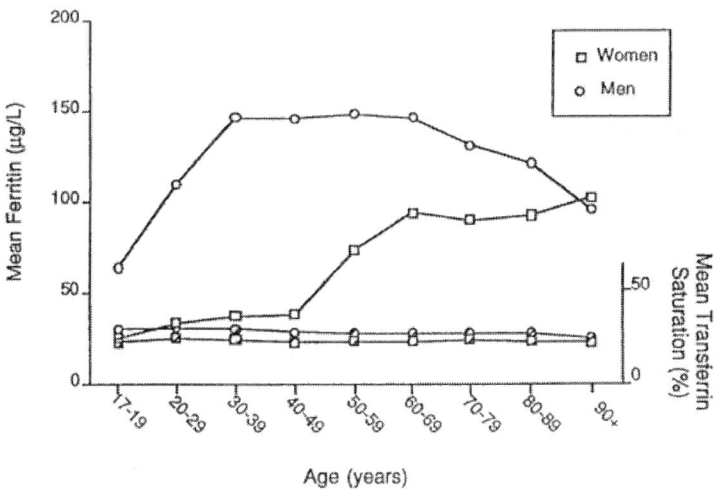

Distribution of serum ferritin level in micrograms per liter and transferrin saturation (%) by decade of age for women and men.

Fertile (pre-menopausal) women lose blood through menstruation, an average of 35 ml a month (though up to 60 is considered normal) or 420 ml a year, and this keeps their iron levels low, since blood is rich in iron, containing the majority of the body's store of it.

Ferritin, a protein that binds iron, is the most common laboratory measure of iron status. Fertile women have average ferritin levels of around 35 ng/ml, while men in the same age range are much higher, around 150. See the chart above.[15]

After they are fully grown, at around the age of 18, men begin to accumulate iron, such that in the following couple of decades, their body iron triples, on average.

At age 45, men have about four times the amount of iron in their bodies as women do, and they also have about four times the rate of heart attacks.

As women reach menopause and cease monthly menstruation, their iron levels rise, and their rates of disease rise also. On average, however, their iron never reaches the levels of men.

The chart (p. 28) shows that average iron levels in men decline starting in the decade of their sixties, and reach a level of around 90 at age 90. This can be attributed to **the faster death rate of men with high iron levels and the greater survival of those men with lower iron levels**. Men with high iron drop out of the population, and thus the averages. The amount of iron in each man doesn't change much, only the average in all men.

Men suffer greater rates of cancer, heart disease, and brain-degenerative disorders like Parkinson's and Alzheimer's than women. Iron is implicated in all of these maladies.

It used to be thought that the hormone estrogen in women protected them from heart disease, and that this was the source of the difference in rates of this disease between men and women. But when women undergo a hysterectomy – thus losing the ability to lose iron through the menstrual cycle – heart disease rates increase, and hormone replacement therapy does not affect this.[16]

If less iron in their bodies explains why women live many years longer than men, as it likely does wholly or partially, that's a very big deal. Iron could represent one of the greatest factors in health, and preventing iron accumulation or lowering high iron stores could be among the most important things anyone could do for their health.

Blood donors are much healthier than non-donors

Since blood is the main storage tissue for iron, containing about 80% of total body iron, loss of blood means loss of iron. Blood donors by definition lose blood, so on average they have lower levels of iron than non-donors.

Several scientific studies have looked at the health of blood donors and found huge health benefits to giving blood.

An issue in studies like these is a bias or selection effect: blood donors on average are likelier to be healthier than non-donors before they ever even donate, since they can't be accepted if they have certain medical conditions, nor would they be as likely to volunteer to donate if they felt unwell. But there are various ways of getting around this limitation, to see whether blood donors are healthier to begin with, whether donating blood makes them healthier, or a combination of both.

Among a group of nearly 3,000 Finnish men, 153 of them had donated blood at least once in the 24 months preceding the start of the study. The entire group was followed for an average of nine years. In that time, one (0.7%) of the donors had a heart attack, while 316 (12.5%) of the non-donor men had a heart attack. After adjusting for age and all the cardiac risk factors they could think of (cholesterol, weight, etc.), the researchers found that **blood donors had an 88% reduced risk of heart attack**.[17]

This study tried to adjust for a healthy donor effect by factoring in standard cardiac risk markers, although there might be additional factors that weren't considered.

In an American population of both men and women who were 40 years old or older and followed for cardiovascular events, those who had donated blood were *half* as likely to have an event such as a heart attack or stroke.[18] All subjects in this study, both donors and non-donors, had no cardiovascular disease at the start of the study.

To get around the healthy donor effect, some studies have compared frequent blood donors to infrequent donors. In one such study, those who had given blood at least once in each of three consecutive years were compared to people who only gave blood one time during the same period. In the following ten years, frequent donors were 40% less likely to have a cardiac event as were infrequent donors.[19]

Another group of researchers compared blood donors to healthy former blood donors to try to account for the healthy donor effect, and they found that each additional annual blood donation was associated with a 7.5% decreased risk of dying in any given period of time.[20] Taken to a logical conclusion, someone who donated blood six times a year – the maximum allowable – would have a 45% lower chance than a non-donor of dying in any given period of time.

This particular study likely *greatly underestimates the health benefits of donating blood,* since the healthy former donors would on average have lower iron levels than non-donors; therefore, the study compares people currently lowering their iron through blood donation to people who previously lowered their iron stores through blood donation. Since iron accumulation occurs slowly, on a scale of years, people who had donated blood in the past will on average have lower iron than those who never donated. When compared to people who have never donated blood, the better health of donors would be even more evident, as we saw above in other studies of blood donation. In effect, this study overcompensates for healthy donor bias.

The data on blood donors provides compelling evidence that lowering iron lowers health risks. When disease-free donors and disease-free non-donors are followed for the same length of time, the donors are much less likely to become ill or to die, even taking the healthy donor effect into account.

Iron levels are related to total mortality

The Copenhagen City Heart Study has studied thousands of residents of that city for many years, and is similar to the Framingham Study in the United States. One research group looked at the study's data on almost 9000 people to determine the relation between ferritin (iron) and death rates.[21]

They found that "stepwise increasing concentrations of ferritin were associated with a stepwise increased risk of premature death overall". People with a ferritin of greater than 600 (a high number) had a median survival age of 55, meaning that of those who had a ferritin that high, half were dead by that age.

Those with a ferritin of 400 to 599 lived an average of 72 years; at 200 to 399, 76 years, and if the ferritin was less than 200, 79 years.

These are startling numbers. Keep in mind that excess iron alone has no symptoms, so many people are walking around with a high ferritin level and don't know it, since only the lab test shows whether someone has high iron or not.

In the Copenhagen study, 26% of men had ferritin levels greater than 200, while only 6% of women did. The death rate increased from 10 to 15% (depending on cause of death) for every 100-point increase in ferritin.

Although this study didn't calculate it, because of the step-wise increase in mortality, I would expect to find that mortality rates decrease at even lower levels of ferritin, e.g. someone with a ferritin of 100 lives longer than someone with a 200 level, and someone with a level of 50 lives even longer.

Junk iron accumulates as we age

One of the biological hallmarks of aging is the accumulation of cellular "junk", which causes damage and poor function.

When young, our cells use a regulated process, autophagy, to clear away old and damaged structures and molecules. As we age, this process declines, so that older people have much lower levels of this process. Fasting and certain substances like resveratrol strongly increase autophagy.

Iron creates the toxic waste of aging

In consequence, the cells of older people accumulate large amounts of junk. The most important kind of junk is called lipofuscin, which has been termed "the toxic waste of aging".

With some exceptions, lipofuscin cannot be degraded, and its association with age is so strong that scientists consider it a reliable marker of the age of both cells and people. As the amount of lipofuscin grows, it impedes important cell functions, leading to a "garbage catastrophe" - so much accumulated trash that nothing works properly.

Many scientists believe that targeting lipofuscin for clearance is an important way to counteract aging and make cells younger.

Iron is a key player in the formation of lipofuscin.[22]

1. Iron builds up in cells
2. Hydrogen peroxide reacts with iron to form lipofuscin
3. Lipofuscin is almost undegradable

4. Lipofuscin decreases autophagic capacity
5. This leads to the accumulation of damaged structures and proteins

Free iron, which is iron that's not locked down by ferritin or other iron storage molecules, is the type that causes damage. The amount of free iron is a function of the amount of total iron, so the less iron in the system altogether, the lower the rate of lipofuscin formation.

Lipofuscin and the iron in it are huge sources of oxidants and can lead to cells becoming senescent, which is a major problem in aging organisms, as the presence of senescent cells causes a system-wide increase in oxidative stress, that is, an overabundance of damaging free radicals, which is a prime characteristic of aging.

Senescent cells are loaded with iron, as much as ten times more than younger, better-functioning cells.

When senescent cells are removed from animals using certain drugs, the animals have much better health and live up to 25% longer.

Poorly functioning mitochondria, the cellular structures often called the powerhouses of the cell, can lead to a cell becoming senescent.[23] Iron accumulation in mitochondria makes them function poorly.[24]

Decreasing the amount of iron in the body should be effective in preventing the formation of lipofuscin and of senescent cells. If these senescent cells are as important to aging and health as some scientists believe, preventing their formation by keeping iron low could be a huge step in fighting aging.

Growth hormone, fasting, and iron

Scientists believe that one of the ways that calorie restriction slows aging is by reducing the amount of growth hormone, which has been implicated in aging and disease.

Growth hormone is, as its name implies, a growth factor, and there is a fundamental trade-off between growth and aging. The bigger and faster an organism grows, the faster it ages.

Iron is also a growth factor. Growing animals, including humans, need iron to help make blood, muscle, and other important physiological components.

Growth hormone increases the uptake of iron from food. This makes sense, since when growth hormone signals the body, it wants to grow, and iron is required for growth.

Growth hormone increases iron by decreasing the amount of another hormone, hepcidin, which controls iron uptake from food. When growth hormone was given to human volunteers, it reduced hepcidin concentrations by about two thirds.[25]

Fasting (going without food for some period of time) retards aging, just as calorie restriction does. Fasting, in contrast to growth hormone, increases the hormone hepcidin, which means that uptake of iron from food decreases.

In short, growth signals cause increased iron uptake and faster aging, and anti-growth signals cause lower iron uptake and slower aging.

So is it growth itself that causes faster aging, or is it the increased iron from growth that does so? Many of the ill effects of human growth hormone supplementation could be due to the accumulation of iron.

Growth – and growth hormone – also promote aging by activating mTOR, a cellular mechanism crucial to growth, and which also plays a major role in aging. The anti-aging drug rapamycin, which extends life in lab animals, works by deactivating mTOR. However, substances which bind and remove iron (chelators) also deactivate mTOR.[26] The deactivation of mTOR is prevented by adding iron.

Less iron = lower mTOR activation = longer life and better health.

Exercise lowers iron

Exercise is known to be one of the most effective health interventions available, and it dramatically lowers the risk of heart disease, cancer, diabetes, dementia, frailty, and a host of other illnesses.

Many of the health benefits of exercise may be connected to its effect on lowering iron.

Athletes are more likely to suffer from iron deficiency, and this does not seem to be due to diet or excess loss of iron, but to a change in iron uptake.

In the days after a race, marathon runners have a nearly three-fold increase in the iron-regulatory hormone hepcidin. The researchers who found this wrote, "the frequently observed iron deficiency of female runners is caused by elevated hepcidin levels."[27]

Lesser amounts of exercise than marathon running also cause elevated levels of hepcidin after exercise.[28] However, whether low-intensity exercises such as walking affect hepcidin and thus iron does not seem to be known.

As we've seen in this section, many factors that affect aging and health are connected to iron. The fact that they affect iron is probably not the whole story about their health benefits, but is likely very important.

Takeaway Points

In this chapter, we've seen that

- calorie restriction, a proven anti-aging intervention, lowers iron levels
- preventing iron accumulation in animals makes them live longer
- healthful plant compounds, such as quercetin and the substances in green tea, lower iron levels
- women live longer than men, and also have lower iron levels
- blood donors, who have lower iron levels, are healthier than non-donors
- in humans, higher iron (ferritin) associates with a higher death rate
- the accumulation of cellular junk is involved in aging, and this junk is loaded with iron
- fasting and exercise, which improve health and increase lifespan, lower iron, while growth hormone, which increases aging, also increases iron
- in short, there's an iron angle to all kinds of healthy interventions as well as states of ill health and of aging. Iron is close to being the universal health mechanism.

2: Iron and Heart Disease

Coronary heart disease is a major scourge in the modern world, and is the leading cause of death in the U.S., killing some 600,000 people annually. As noted in the first chapter, men have much greater rates of heart disease than women, and men die of heart disease at rates from two- to five-fold higher than women. Why is this?

For a long time, it was thought that the difference was in sex hormones, which obviously differ greatly between men and women. Either female sex hormones like estrogen were protective, or male hormones like testosterone caused harm. That was the thinking anyway, and some still do think this.

But in 1981, Dr. Jerome Sullivan, a pathologist, first proposed that the difference between men and women in heart disease risk was due to iron in the body, of which men have much more than women.

In the Framingham Study, which studied a large group of people for many years, it was found that both natural menopause and hysterectomy increased the risk of heart disease in women. Therefore, the answer to the increased rate of heart disease in men cannot be hormones.[29]

The chart below shows the difference in rates of coronary heart disease by age, sex, and menopausal status.[30]

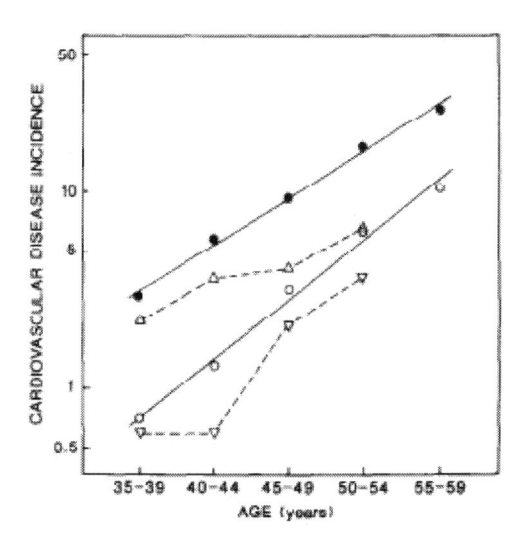

Figure 1: Incidence of heart disease by age and sex. From lowest to highest: fertile women, all women, post-menopausal women, and men.

Men have higher rates of heart disease at any age, and post-menopausal women have much higher rates than pre-menopausal women, even at the same age. Hormone replacement therapy with estrogen does not protect post-menopausal women from heart disease.

Women who use the birth control pill have both higher iron levels and higher rates of heart disease.

Pre-menopausal women lose blood through their menstrual cycle, an average of about 35 milliliters a month, or about 420 milliliters a year. Since blood is the major storage tissue for iron, containing about 80% of the body's total, losing blood means losing iron. And in fact, pre-menopausal women do have much less iron in their bodies.

What about cholesterol? Haven't we been told for a long time to lower it and that it causes heart attacks? To see whether this is true take a look at the following chart:

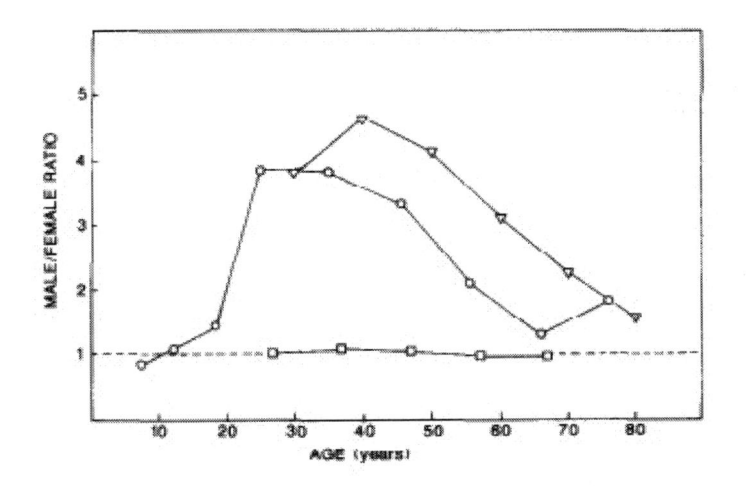

Figure 2: Effect of age on sex ratio of heart disease deaths (inverted triangles), sex ratio of serum ferritin (circles), sex ratio of cholesterol (squares).

The chart shows the sex ratio in heart disease deaths by age, that is, the number of men divided by the number of women who have heart disease at any age. Also plotted is the sex ratio of the median ferritin (iron) level by age. Finally, at the bottom of the graph is the sex ratio of total cholesterol by age.

Cholesterol hardly matters. Men have both much higher ferritin levels than women, and a much higher rate of death from heart disease.

Among men alone, that is, comparing men only to other men, greater iron means more heart attacks. Men with a ferritin (a measure of iron) greater than 200, after adjusting for a host of factors, including age, cigarette pack-years, abnormal ECG in an exercise test, maximal oxygen uptake, systolic blood pressure, blood glucose, serum copper, HDL cholesterol, and triglyceride concentrations, had 2.2 times the risk of a heart attack than did those with ferritin less than 200.[31]

Many, many men have a ferritin of 200 or more. Not a single laboratory even considers 200 to be abnormal. Your doctor doesn't consider 200 to be abnormal. (We'll discuss what is normal or abnormal for iron later on.)

Heart attacks show a strong circadian variation, and are three times more likely to occur at 9:00 A.M. than at 11:00 P.M. This pattern coincides with the variation in serum iron levels, which are two to three times higher in the morning than at night.

Carotid artery disease is another form of cardiovascular disease that greatly raises the risk of stroke, and happens when plaque builds up and narrows the opening of the arteries. The biological mechanism that causes this is similar to that which causes coronary artery disease. As ferritin (iron) increases, so does the risk of carotid artery disease. See the chart below.

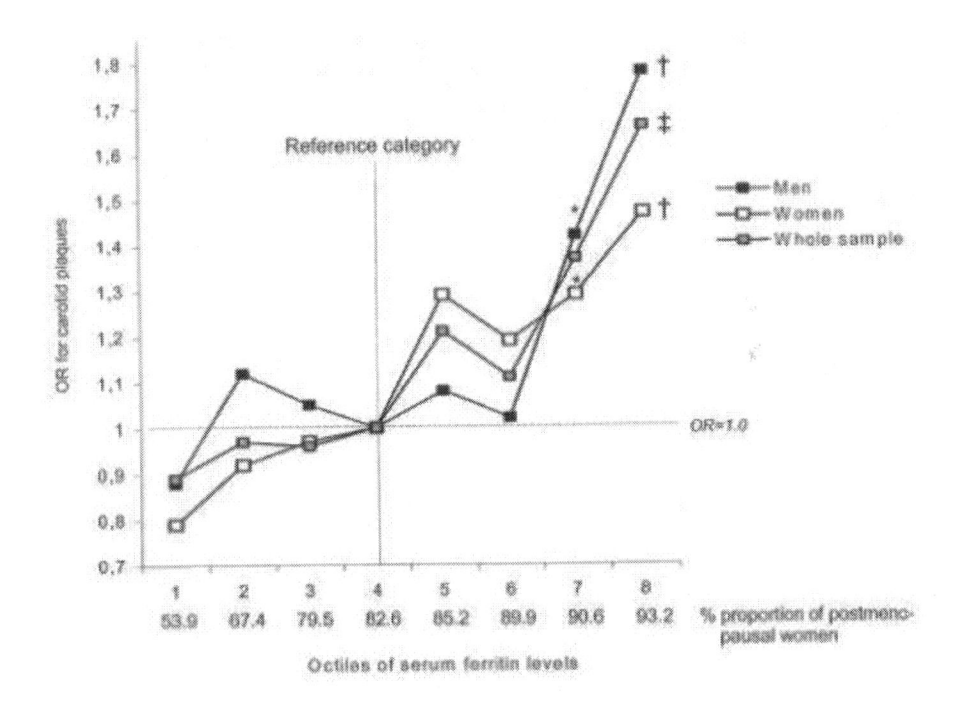

How does iron block arteries? Iron is highly reactive, and can damage lipids and other molecules, causing inflammation that leads to arterial plaque. Iron is increased in atherosclerotic lesions as compared with normal arterial walls.

Low iron also increases nitric oxide, an important factor in the protection of the walls of blood vessels.[32]

Statin drugs, iron and heart disease

Statin drugs can reduce the risk of heart disease, and it's widely thought that this is due to their influence on cholesterol. However, pre-menopausal women are largely protected from heart disease, regardless of their cholesterol levels. Hormone replacement therapy (HRT) in post-menopausal women improves lipid profiles, but fails to protect against atherosclerosis or heart attacks. Something besides cholesterol is causing heart disease.

Statins affect iron metabolism by clearing free iron. The use of statins is also associated with lower ferritin (iron) levels.[33]

In a study that lowered iron via phlebotomy, some of the patients were taking statins. It was found that improved health outcomes were associated with lower ferritin values, but not with improved cholesterol (HDL and LDL).[34]

Iron looks like a much more promising candidate as causative of heart disease than cholesterol.

Less wealthy countries outside the West also have much lower rates of coronary heart disease than in the West. The people in them also eat diets that are lower in iron, they have lower body iron stores, and iron deficiency is more common. Variation in heart disease rates between countries are strongly correlated to body iron stores.[35]

The evidence that heart attacks are related to iron comes from disparate sources: experiments using lab animals or cell cultures, and epidemiological studies of the general population or of blood donors.

As iron levels go up with age, the risk of heart attack also increases. Men have greater heart disease risk than women, and post-menopausal women greater risk than pre-menopausal. Iron damages arterial walls. Combine all of these and there's a clear case for the relation of excess iron to coronary heart disease.

Takeaway Points

- The difference between men and women in heart disease risk is, at least in part, due to higher iron levels in men
- In men alone, those with higher iron have more heart disease
- In women, menopause results in both higher iron

levels and rising rates of heart disease

- In fertile (pre-menopausal) women, monthly blood loss means lower iron levels than men, along with much lower risk of heart attack
- High iron levels are associated with carotid artery plaque
- Statins may work through their effect on iron
- Variation in heart disease rates by country are related to iron stores
- Iron is a highly reactive metal and can damage arterial walls

3: Iron Causes Cancer

To lower your risk of cancer, you must take control of your iron.

The incidence of cancer increases with age, and as we've seen, so do iron levels.

Men have higher rates of both cancer and death from cancer than women, and they also have higher iron levels. For some forms of cancer, the risk for men is up to four-fold higher than for women.[36] Overall, men have around a 35% higher risk of dying from cancer than women. Higher body iron stores in men could explain much of this difference, since men start to accumulate iron after the age of 18, whereas most women do not accumulate excess iron until after age 50.[37]

The most striking evidence that iron is involved with cancer comes from a study in which a group of patients were randomized either to phlebotomy (bloodletting) in order to lower their iron levels, or to no treatment.[38] The patients were part of a study designed to test whether phlebotomy could treat peripheral arterial disease, and they had no cancer at the start of the study. They were followed for an average of 4.5 years.

Results showed that those patients assigned to iron-reduction had a 35% decreased rate of cancer, and an approximately 60% reduced rate of death from cancer, compared to those who had no iron-reduction treatment.

Furthermore, phlebotomy doesn't make iron levels the same in all people. The level of iron depends on the starting point – those with higher iron levels at the beginning require more phlebotomy to lower iron than do those who have a lower iron level to start with. The iron level also depends on compliance with their treatment, that is, those who consistently show up for their appointments and get their blood drawn and thus have more withdrawn overall end up with lower iron than people who show up less or not at all.

Therefore, it's important to note that in this study, those who developed cancer in either the iron-reduction or no-treatment groups had similar and higher levels of iron, but those who did not develop cancer, in either group, had much lower levels of iron. Ferritin (iron) in those who developed cancer averaged 127 ng/ml, while in those that remained cancer free, ferritin was 76.

As we'll see later in this book, it's relatively easy to attain an iron level similar to the group that did not develop cancer. It's also relatively easy to have a level similar to the group that did develop it, if you have a standard Western lifestyle and don't actively do anything about your iron.

A population study found that people with high iron levels, using a cutoff value, had 3 times the risk of colon cancer and 1.5 times the risk of lung cancer.[39]

Researchers in Taiwan found that men who were at the high end of the normal range for iron levels, as compared to the low end, had about a 3-fold increase in cancer rates.[40]

A population study of over 6000 American men and women, who were free of cancer at the beginning of the study, found that those in the highest quartile (fourth) of serum iron had almost *double* the risk of dying from cancer.[41] Noteworthy, at all levels of iron, the men had a cancer death rate of 4.7 per 1000 person-years, while for women it was much lower at 2.8. Iron strikes again.

Iron chelators fight cancer

If iron causes cancer, then we would expect to find that iron chelators, synthetic or natural chemicals that bind and remove iron, would lower cancer rates or perhaps even treat cancer.

That is in fact what we do find. In lab mice that are implanted with prostate cancer cells, the iron chelator IP6, found in rice bran, reduced the growth of tumors by 75% when added to their drinking water.[42]

In another study done in mice, iron chelators had remarkably potent anti-tumor activity, shrinking tumors in mice by half in only five days. The effect of these chelators was comparable to the anti-cancer chemotherapy drug doxorubicin.[43] The iron chelators activate a cellular pathway that leads to self-destruction in cancer cells. Their activity left normal cells, including blood and immune cells, untouched.

There are many other, similar studies, both on lab animals and in cell culture.

What about in humans?

A research study set out to find if they could prevent cancer in a group at high-risk. Men who had a prostate condition, prostate neoplasia, that gives them a high risk of cancer, were divided into two groups. Thirty men took green tea extract capsules, 200 mg each, three times a day, for a year. Another thirty men took a placebo capsule. The compounds in green tea extract are strong iron chelators.

After a year, 30% of the men in the placebo group were diagnosed with cancer. In the green tea extract group, only one man, or about 3%, developed cancer. The risk reduction was 90% - a startling result.

These compounds, the catechins in green tea extract (in the human study) and IP6 (in the mouse study), have a number of other effects on cells besides the removal of iron, so we can't be sure that the iron chelating effect was the cause, or the sole cause, of their cancer-fighting ability. Still, other compounds whose only function is the chelating of iron have been shown effective against cancer cells, and they have been suggested for use in cancer treatment.[44]

Aspirin lowers both iron and cancer rates

Recently it's been found that long-term use of low-dose aspirin results in a significant decrease in cancer rates, as much as 75% lower in the case of esophageal cancer.[45] Other cancers saw 30 to 50% lower rates, and overall, aspirin users had about 20% lower rates of cancer. Since aspirin lowers inflammation, some have speculated that this could be the mechanism of aspirin's anti-cancer effects.

Others have made the connection with iron. Aspirin, even in low doses, causes small amounts of bleeding from the intestines, usually not enough to be detectable. But this bleeding, if it goes on long enough, results in lower iron levels among aspirin users.

Long-term use of low-dose aspirin results in a cumulative reduction in iron, similar to what can be achieved by phlebotomy. This mechanism is compatible with the observation that the effect of low-dose aspirin on cancer doesn't kick in until about five years of aspirin use.

Aspirin is also associated with a much lower risk of metastasis, which is the spread of the cancer to distant body sites from the original tumor.[46] Long-term use of low-dose aspirin reduced the risk of metastasis by up to 75% in the case of colon cancer, and up to 50% in other cancers. Again, depriving tumors access to iron may be an important mechanism in the reduction of metastases.

I'll discuss aspirin further in the section on lowering iron levels.

Smoking, iron, and lung cancer

Curiously, current American cigarette smokers have a risk of lung cancer far higher, as much as ten times higher, than current Japanese smokers.[47] This shows that other, perhaps multiple factors, affect the risk of lung cancer besides smoking.

Aspirin is one factor that can reduce the risk of lung cancer. Men who had a history of aspirin use had about a 26% lower risk of lung cancer. But aspirin showed no effect in women.[48] This fact may strengthen the case for iron's involvement in lung cancer, since women have lower iron levels than men. Lowering those levels further with aspirin had no effect; but lowering the higher iron levels of men lowered their risk of lung cancer.

Iron and Cancer Stem Cells

Cancer stem cells are cancer cells found within a tumor that are capable of differentiating into other cancer cells. They appear to be an important source not only of tumors, but of recurrence of cancer after therapy; that is, cancer stem cells must be wiped out entirely to prevent the recurrence of the disease. Therapy fails if cancer stem cells remain, and these cells are also important in metastasis.

Iron induces cancer stem cells when the iron is at normal, physiological (i.e. non-toxic) levels.[49] Iron up-regulates certain genes in cancer stem cells, and as such iron plays an important role in "aggressive cancer behaviors" and metastasis.

Conversely, control of iron represents a therapeutic target of cancer stem cells.[50] Iron added to a cell culture of cancer stem cells strongly promoted their growth, but iron chelators, chemicals that bind and remove iron, suppressed their growth. The lower the iron in the cell medium, the fewer cancer stem cells.

The authors of this study concluded, "Iron is a key element for the proliferation and differentiation of cancer stem cells. Iron controlling therapy including iron chelators is a novel therapeutic target of cancer stem cells."

Keeping iron levels in a low normal range should be a sound anti-cancer intervention.

Cancer as a ferrotoxic disease

Some scientists have been explicit in the relation between iron and cancer, saying that cancer has aspects of a "ferrotoxic disease".[51] In plain language, that means that iron can cause cancer. Indeed, iron is carcinogenic in lab animals, and many conditions of iron-overload in humans are associated with higher risks of cancer.

Shinya Toyokuni, one such scientist, has said that "fine control of body iron stores would be a wise strategy for cancer prevention".

In other words, knowing your iron level and controlling it can help prevent cancer. Many people can easily tell you their cholesterol number, since doctors like to measure it often, and the media tells us how important it is. But almost no one knows their iron level, which in the estimation of this writer and that of many others, is far more important for health than cholesterol.

That needs to change.

The link between iron and cancer is underrated

There are a number of other studies that could be cited on the relation between iron levels and cancer, but let's stop with these. The reason for citing studies at the risk of boring the reader is because in mainstream health and fitness writing, how often do you hear that excess iron may cause cancer?

Never. That's how often.

Have you ever heard your doctor mention the cancer risks of too much iron? For 99.9% of readers, the answer is surely "no".

The common belief about cancer is that, except for the case of smoking and lung cancer, it somehow just appears and there's nothing much anyone can do about it. Cancer is often treated as a literal tragedy, a fate which strikes at random or a destiny which can't be avoided.

That is just not the case. While iron is not the only thing that causes cancer or increases its risk, it's an important cause, especially among otherwise healthy people who appear to have few other risk factors.

Even with smoking and cancer, the high concentration of iron in tobacco smoke means that iron could be one of its most important cancer-causing components.[52]

How iron causes cancer

Iron causes the formation of harmful free radicals, particularly the hydroxyl radical, and this can interact with cell structures and damage them. Among the structures damaged is DNA, and mutations in DNA can lead to cancer.[53] DNA damage can be prevented with iron chelators – chemicals that bind and remove iron.

Cancer cells are characterized by uncontrolled growth and make high demands on a number of nutrients, notably glucose and iron, so once cancer has been initiated, iron can fuel its growth. In mice, tumors grow twice as fast when fed a normal iron as opposed to a low iron diet.

Another way that iron can promote cancer is by suppressing immune function. Normally, the cells of the immune system monitor the body for cancer cells, and destroy them when encountered. Failure of immunity is therefore crucial in cancer development, and too much iron can cause a decrease in immune cell function. Cancer cells then either escape detection or cannot be destroyed.

So to avoid cancer, keeping iron levels low will help, and we'll discuss how to do that and what level of iron you should target in a later chapter.

If you don't smoke, don't drink alcohol to excess, exercise, avoid processed foods, stay lean, and get enough vitamin D, you may think you've done everything in your power to stay healthy and avoid cancer. Unfortunately, that's not the case, because if you have a high iron level, that's an important risk factor you haven't touched.

Takeaway points

- Men have both higher iron stores than women and higher risk of cancer
- Phlebotomy (bloodletting) dramatically lowers the risk of cancer
- Men or women with high ferritin (iron) levels have greater risk of cancer
- Iron chelators fight cancer
- Aspirin lowers the risk of cancer, and also lowers iron stores
- Cancer cells require large amounts of iron
- Iron fuels tumor growth

4: Iron Is Linked to Brain Diseases and Cognitive Decline

Alzheimer's disease, Parkinson's disease, and dementia rank among the most dreaded diseases of old age. People fear them so much not because they are literally worse than, say, cancer, but because they seem to rob us of our identity. By causing the decline of brain function, our very selves melt away, until we're left helpless and a burden to others.

Brain iron and Alzheimer's disease

Alzheimer's disease is perhaps the most well-known brain disorder. In this illness, the neurons in the brain become loaded with plaques that inhibit functioning.

Iron is intimately involved in the pathogenesis of Alzheimer's. High concentrations of iron are found in the plaques that characterize this disease.[54] Furthermore, the accumulation of iron in the parts of the brain that are affected by Alzheimer's correlates with damage.[55]

Oxidative stress, that is, an excess of free radicals that

causes damage, is strongly associated with Alzheimer's disease.[56] Excess iron causes oxidative stress, providing a further mechanistic link.

Type 2 diabetes, which is characterized by insulin resistance, is a risk factor for Alzheimer's, and in fact this disease has been called "type 3 diabetes". Diabetes can result in deregulation of iron metabolism leading to excess iron accumulation in the brain.

According to a group that studied Alzheimer's, "A *consistent* observation in AD is a dysregulation of metal ions", including iron. Note the word "consistent", which fingers iron as a cause. They propose that iron-chelating compounds, including EGCG from green tea, and curcumin, are promising therapeutic agents for Alzheimer's.[57]

Iron (ferritin) as measured in spinal fluid is independently associated with cognitive decline leading to Alzheimer's. The levels of ferritin can actually predict cognitive status.[58] One reason this result is important is because it shows that the level of the allegedly safe-storage form of iron, ferritin, is strongly associated with cognitive decline: more ferritin, more decline. It doesn't look like ferritin is so safe after all. The researchers believe that the excess brain iron in Alzheimer's has a genetic basis, and while it may very well have such a basis, iron must come from outside the body, and it can be inhibited or removed by several methods – which we'll be discussing later.

Men have higher rates of Alzheimer's, and in healthy older men, common gene variants that control iron metabolism were associated with increased levels of iron in the brain.[59] Men generally also have higher levels of brain iron than do women, explaining men's higher risk of Alzheimer's and other brain diseases.

A group of scientists recently reported a startling discovery: when they looked at brains of ten Alzheimer's patients, they found fungi in every one of them, and they found zero fungi in ten patients without the disease.[60] As we'll see in the section on infections, fungi require iron to grow and reproduce; so excess iron in the brain could be providing the fuel for these microorganisms, leading to Alzheimer's. In this scenario, iron chelators or phlebotomy could deprive fungi or other microbial invaders of iron, leading to their demise. The fungal infection hypothesis here fits well with the slow progression of the disease, as well as immune system activation seen in it.

Brain iron, Parkinson's disease, and lifespan

Parkinson's disease is a progressive brain disorder that affects movement. Its cause is the loss of neurons that produce dopamine in the substantia nigra, a region of the midbrain. Oxidative damage causes the death of these neurons.

Parkinson's, if not treated properly, can be fatal.

According to Joseph Knoll, the Hungarian discoverer of the drug selegiline (Deprenyl), which is used to treat Parkinson's, all humans lose on average 13% of their dopamine neurons per decade after the age of 45. This loss appears central to the process of aging.

At that rate, if we lived long enough, everyone would develop Parkinson's. The reason why some people develop Parkinson's and others do not is because they lose neurons at a rate greater than 13% a decade. When dopamine neurons decline in number to about 30% of normal, the disease sets in, and when these neurons decline to 10% of

THE AGE-RELATED DECLINE OF STRIATAL DOPAMINE IN HUMANS

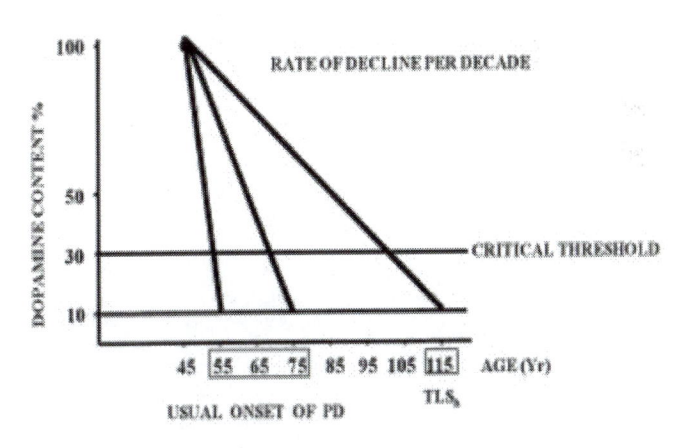

normal, death occurs.

The chart above, taken from Knoll's book, shows that with a steeper rate of decline of dopamine neurons, Parkinson's occurs between the ages of 55 and 75, and that with a "normal" rate of decline, death from Parkinson's would occur for everyone at the age of 115. The decline in numbers of dopamine neurons sets a limit to human lifespan.

Deprenyl, the drug that Knoll discovered, both protects dopamine neurons from destruction and extends the lifespan of lab animals, which lends additional support to the theory that dopamine neurons set a limit on lifespan. In Knoll's study on rats, those on Deprenyl lived 35% longer than controls. That's a huge extension, comparable to calorie restriction.

Parkinson's disease is also associated with the accumulation of iron in the parts of the brain that this disease affects.[61]

Besides extending lifespan in lab animals, Deprenyl protects the brain against excess iron.[62] This means that iron causes the death of dopamine neurons and that protecting them from iron both protects against Parkinson's disease and decreases aging. Protecting the brain from the accumulation of excess iron is crucial for good brain health in older age as well as for life extension.

Men have higher rates of both Parkinson's and Alzheimer's, and men also accumulate more iron in the affected regions of the brain.[63] Men also have higher levels of iron overall. Aging is also strongly associated with both diseases, and older people have more iron in their bodies than younger people.

Mild cognitive impairment, a precursor to Alzheimer's, is also characterized by iron accumulation in the brain.[64]

Many researchers have noted the connection between iron accumulation and brain disorders, and have therefore suggested therapies based on removing the iron. One review article suggested phlebotomy, the targeted removal of blood and lowering of iron stores, as a therapy for Alzheimer's.[65] A quote from the article summary:

> "Body iron stores that increase with age could be pivotal to AD [Alzheimer's disease] pathogenesis and progression. Increased stored iron is associated with common medical conditions such as diabetes and vascular disease that increase risk for development of AD. Increased stored iron could also promote oxidative stress/free radical damage in vulnerable neurons, a critical early change in AD. A ferrocentric model of AD described here forms the basis of a rational, easily testable experimental therapeutic approach for AD, which if successful, would be both widely applicable and inexpensive. Clinical studies have shown that calibrated phlebotomy is an effective way to reduce stored iron safely and predictably without causing anemia. We hypothesize that reducing stored iron by calibrated phlebotomy to avoid iron deficiency will improve cerebrovascular function, slow neurodegenerative change, and improve cognitive and behavioral functions in AD."

Iron chelators, which are drugs or other natural chemicals that bind to iron and remove it, have also been suggested for both Alzheimer's and Parkinson's.

Catechins, which are substances found in green tea, have also been suggested as treatments for these brain diseases. These substances chelate iron and cross the blood-brain barrier, penetrating the brain to remove iron.[66]

Ferritin: dynamite in storage

At this point, let's digress a bit into the issue of free iron versus ferritin.

As noted, iron is a highly reactive atom, much like oxygen, and therefore the body has developed mechanisms for controlling its reactivity, for "locking it down" behind protective molecular walls, so that it becomes safer and less likely to do damage. The principal means that the body has for controlling iron is the protein molecule ferritin, which sequesters iron atoms in its core and makes them unavailable for reaction with other molecules.

Each ferritin molecule stores up to 4,500 iron atoms inside it.

As we age, ferritin levels tend to increase, reflecting the increase in iron stores that result from continued ingestion of iron and, in most cases, very little loss.

Also as we age, there's a tendency for free iron to increase. Essentially, the body becomes worse at being able to lock iron down with ferritin, and the amount of free iron in the system increases. This is an unhealthy situation.

In many or most cases of disease, such as in Alzheimer's and Parkinson's, the culprit doing the damage is free iron, not ferritin, or at least that's the current thinking. (Much remains to be learned about both iron metabolism and brain diseases.) Therefore, the question arises as to whether lowering ferritin levels through phlebotomy will help decrease the risks of disease, or treat diseases when already present.

Part of the problem in Alzheimer's and Parkinson's may be due to disordered iron regulation. In other words, there may be something about the physiology of the brain in patients with those diseases that disposes it to higher levels of free iron. Factors that favor higher free iron could be genetic or environmental, or both.

Nevertheless, higher brain levels of ferritin, the iron-storage molecule, are also seen in patients with these diseases. Just having enough ferritin around is enough to trigger the release of free iron, which then causes damage.

Excessive ferritin can be compared to having a box full of dynamite in your house; it's safe enough if that dynamite never gets near fire, but it's an accident waiting to happen. So generally, you don't want to keep a box of dynamite at home. The same applies to ferritin. Elevated levels of free radicals inside neurons and glial cells (the supporting cast in the brain) likely cause iron to be released from ferritin, like a match lighting a stick of dynamite.

So, even though ferritin is considered a safe form of iron, lowering its levels through phlebotomy or some other means decreases the amount of damaging free iron. Simply put, less of it is available to explode.

Furthermore, certain treatments can increase the amount of ferritin protein, which is then available for the storage of iron, decreasing the amount of free iron in the system.

Such treatments include substances that cause hormesis, which occurs when the body activates molecular defense systems in reaction to certain stimulatory agents or low-dose toxins. Familiar agents that work through hormesis include EGCG and other substances in green tea, curcumin, resveratrol, and others. Some of these may therefore be useful in preventing or treating Alzheimer's and Parkinson's.

Other interventions that work through hormesis include exercise and intermittent fasting, so staying lean and in shape could go a long way toward preventing the brain diseases of aging by keeping iron metabolism well-regulated. These interventions also greatly decrease the risk of type 2 diabetes, which in turn decreases the risk of Alzheimer's.

Iron chelators' mode of action is to directly interact with free iron, not ferritin, and remove it. IP6 (inositol hexaphosphate), a molecule refined from rice bran, strongly chelates iron and removes it, and it has been suggested as a treatment in Parkinson's.[67] In cell culture, IP6 significantly protects neurons, the cells of the brain.

We'll have much more to say on iron chelators later.

Takeaway points

- Both Alzheimer's and Parkinson's diseases are associated with high iron in the brain
- Parkinson's disease is due to death of dopamine neurons, and this happens to everyone
- Iron is also increased in mild cognitive impairment
- Phlebotomy (bloodletting) may treat Alzheimer's
- Ferritin can be degraded into free iron, which causes damage. It's biological dynamite
- Iron chelators reduce free iron, the damaging kind

5: Diabetes, Obesity, and Iron

We're in the midst of an obesity epidemic, and diabetes is strongly on the rise as a consequence. Could there be an iron connection to both of these? There's lots of evidence that there is.

First, there's an association between iron and obesity. In a group of Japanese people, average age 58, ferritin was significantly correlated with visceral fat, subcutaneous fat, liver fat, and insulin resistance.[68] Similar results were seen in a Mexican population.[69]

Obesity is characterized by insulin resistance, the relative inability of cells to respond properly to insulin, a hormone secreted by the pancreas. Insulin promotes the uptake of glucose (sugar) from the blood into cells, and it prevents the release of fat from fat cells. When insulin resistance goes on long enough, type 2 diabetes can result.

In obesity, iron levels increase, insulin sensitivity and adiponectin levels decline, and excess calories are then shunted to fat cells. This is accompanied by increased inflammation and oxidative stress.

What causes iron levels to increase? For one thing, aging. As we've noted, the body has no regulated way to rid itself of excess iron; bleeding is the only natural way to lower iron stores – and this isn't regulated. The body "wants" to hang on to all the iron it can get, because in evolutionary terms, iron is a scarce resource, and the downside of excess iron usually only occurs at an older age, when evolutionary pressures are relaxed.

Older age is associated with obesity, insulin resistance, oxidative stress, and inflammation – and with excess iron.

Refined carbohydrates such as flour have taken much of the blame for the obesity epidemic, maybe deservedly so. But other countries, such as France and Italy and the Scandinavian countries, eat plenty of foods with flour in them, such as bread and pastries and pasta, and have much less obesity than the U.S. In the U.S., flour is iron-fortified, but not in those other countries. Perhaps iron is the reason for the much greater rate of obesity in the U.S.

Furthermore, a fad (for lack of a better word) for gluten-free products has become strong in recent years, with many people saying that gluten, one of the components of wheat, makes them ill, and having success at curing their ills when they stop eating gluten. Here again, iron may be a factor. As we'll see when we look at infections, bacteria love iron and require it to grow and reproduce. The type of iron added to flour and other refined carbohydrates is free iron, which is instantly available to bacteria, much more so than the iron in meat, which is locked down in the heme molecule. The gut contains billions of bacteria, and feeding them iron could be expected to increase that number as well as change the mix of bacterial species, leading to dysbiosis and gut health problems. Perhaps the real reason that some people feel better when they give up gluten is that they're getting much less iron in their gut, so less is available to feed bacteria, and their gut heals.

Adiponectin

Adiponectin is a hormone that regulates appetite, and also has a number of healthful effects. In obesity, adiponectin declines, and this is thought to be behind some of the illnesses, such as cardiovascular problems and diabetes, associated with obesity.[70]

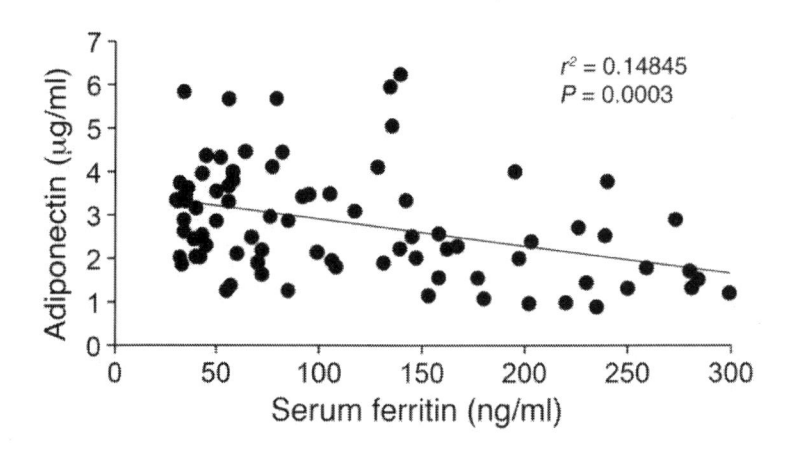

Laboratory animals fed a high-iron diet have decreased adiponectin, and fat cells treated with iron have lower secretion of this hormone. In humans, ferritin (iron in the body) is increased in obese diabetic subjects, and this lowers adiponectin.[71] See chart above.

Phlebotomy (bloodletting) lowers iron stores and increases insulin sensitivity.[72]

In the case of obesity and diabetes, we're faced with a chicken-and-egg problem: which comes first, increased iron leading to obesity and diabetes, or obesity and diabetes leading to increased iron?

The facts on this matter are not firmly established, and it appears to this writer that both of these could be the case depending on the person, or even in the same person. Since getting rid of excess iron leads to better insulin sensitivity, which comes first may not matter, as it may be iron that is causing most of the metabolic damage. In other words, merely by depleting excess iron, or by preventing excess iron in the first place, much of the metabolic damage of obesity may be undone or prevented. Diabetics who do nothing but lower their iron stores may see increased insulin sensitivity, and this may in turn treat or mitigate their diabetes.

Besides creating the metabolic conditions for increased iron, another way to acquire excess iron is through iron-adulterated food. *All flour, corn meal, and rice in the U.S. is required by law to be fortified with iron.*

Our food is poisoning us with iron.

Other sources of iron include multivitamins and iron-fortified breakfast cereals. From 15 to 20% of the adult population in the U.S. take iron supplements.[73] Practically everyone eats cereal.

Certain foods also accelerate iron absorption through regulation of hepcidin, the hormone that controls iron absorption. For instance, eating refined carbohydrates and sugar, which are associated with obesity, alters iron metabolism, leading to increased iron uptake, with the consequent oxidative stress leading to insulin resistance, and then obesity.

But whether eating refined carbohydrates ultimately causes iron levels to increase, or whether iron itself goes up on its own (through eating too much of it), iron causes oxidative stress through reacting with molecules and cellular structures, leading to insulin resistance, decreased adiponectin, and obesity. We can certainly make a case for that scenario.

Some people can eat plenty of carbohydrates and sugar and never get fat, and that can be seen as a refutation of the theory that these nutrients cause obesity. That could be true. But those who can eat these foods and not get fat tend to be young, and the younger a person is, the less likely he is to have high iron stores, and thus better insulin sensitivity and resistance to obesity.

Iron makes you hungry

Iron supplementation increases appetite, so this fact alone provides a mechanism for more iron leading to more food intake with subsequent obesity.

Iron deficiency causes a loss of appetite.

Supplementation and deficiency are two ends of an extreme of iron intake, but even somewhere in the middle, such as eating iron-fortified food – which is hard to avoid in the U.S. - the increase in appetite may be enough to tip the balance into overeating and weight gain.

Ferritin (iron) levels are highly correlated with food intake, i.e. more iron in the body means more food eaten.[74]

Some of the effects of iron on hunger are because it decreases the hormone leptin, which is secreted by fat cells and is known as the satiety hormone.[75] Levels of stored iron (ferritin) are among the best predictors of levels of leptin.

Less leptin means less satiety and more hunger. Leptin levels are negatively correlated with body mass index.

Take a look at the following chart to see the strong correlation between ferritin and leptin. Each point represents a different person.

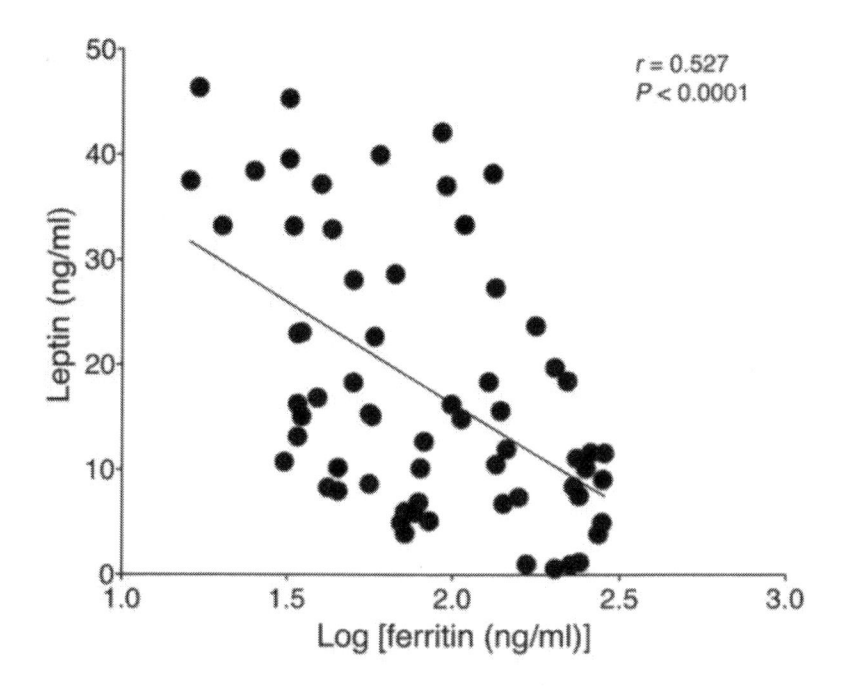

Figure: Scatter plot of Leptin (ng/ml) vs Log[ferritin (ng/ml)], r = 0.527, P < 0.0001.

The ferritin values in the chart were all within the so-called normal range, so these are not extreme cases, but values found in healthy, non-iron-overloaded people. In otherwise healthy people, "normal" levels of iron can vary as much as 15-fold. As we'll see later, there are good reasons to believe that this is not normal at all.

When mice are fed a high-iron diet, their leptin levels decrease due to the effect of iron on fat cells.

Iron affects fat cells and hormones that control eating. More iron means less control of hunger.

So is it possible to lose weight by controlling the level of iron in the body, or by eating less iron from food?

It would be premature to say so, but I consider it probable.

The chart below, from a U.S. government study on nutrients in the American diet, shows that iron consumption has increased dramatically in recent years.[76]

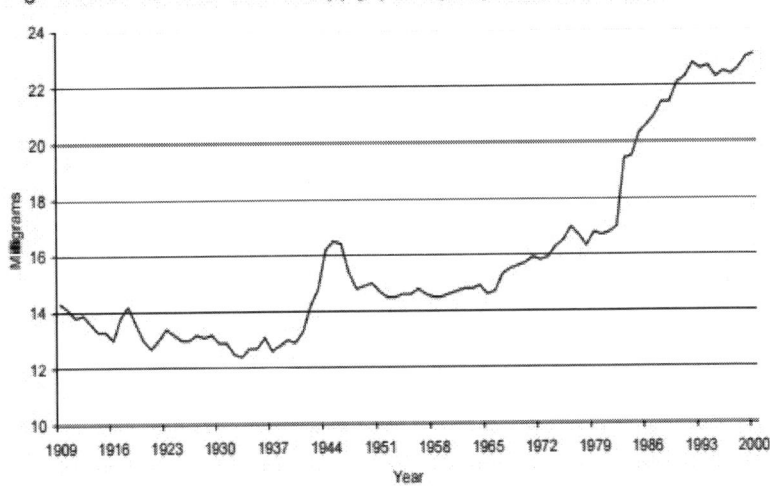

Figure 41. Iron in the U.S. food supply, per capita per day, 1909-2000

Could the huge increase in iron consumption in recent decades have anything to do with the obesity epidemic? If the obesity epidemic started in the early 1970s, then there's certainly quite a coincidence between rising iron intake and the rate of obesity.

Furthermore, sugar has taken much of the blame for the obesity epidemic; consumption of sugar and high-fructose corn syrup has gone up.

Sugar massively increases the uptake of iron by the cells of the intestines.[77] So sugar could lead to a higher iron load in the body, with lost control of hunger, leading to obesity.

If you want to lose weight, checking your body iron (ferritin) level would be a good idea, and if it's too high, steps can be taken to bring it down. The avoidance of high iron foods as well as food and drink that increase iron absorption, e.g. orange juice, is another good step. Certain dietary items such as green tea strongly inhibit iron absorption from food – this may be one of the reasons the Japanese stay slender.

All of this – what constitutes a high iron level, what foods are high in iron, how iron can be inhibited or removed – will be covered in the last chapter of this book.

Takeaway points

- Serum (blood) levels of ferritin are associated with obesity
- Iron causes derangement of hormones that control hunger
- Iron intake has increased dramatically at the same time as obesity has gone up
- Iron supplementation increases hunger; deficiency decreases it

6: Iron is implicated in many other diseases

A feature of a number of other diseases is either iron overload or degraded iron metabolism. Decreasing the iron load of the ill person has either been shown or suggested to treat them. Following are a few of them. I use the word "few" advisedly, since iron is involved in virtually all pathological processes in some way or another.

Infections

Infectious organisms (pathogens), like all other living things, require iron, and have evolved systems to acquire iron in the hosts that they infect.

In the eternal arms race between parasite and host, living things have also evolved ways to withhold iron from microbial invaders.

Most bacterial, all fungal and all protozoan pathogenic invaders require iron as an essential growth factor. Viruses use iron in the host cell for their reproduction, even though they contain no iron themselves. The less iron available for these organisms, the less the likelihood of becoming infected and the less the severity of the illness in case of infection.[78]

Some pathogenic microorganisms invade cells (intracellular pathogens), and are able to acquire iron-containing ferritin molecules for their own purposes. Other pathogens may dissolve tissues and thus obtain the iron in them.[79] Intestinal pathogens such as *Salmonella* grow better when they have more access to iron, and iron supplementation can increase the rate of infection with organisms like these. Malarial infection increases with iron supplements.

Hemodialysis patients who were given supplemental iron had nearly twice the rate of infections as those who were given no iron.[80] Taking extra iron, or having high iron stores, appears to be a good way to get an infection.

Sepsis is a serious and often fatal infection in which bacteria or other organisms invade the bloodstream, and iron is a critical factor in their growth.[81] In experimental sepsis induced in mice, iron greatly exacerbated the sepsis, such that none of the animals with sepsis died, but the combination of iron and sepsis produced a combined 60% rate of death or being moribund (about to die).[82]

Iron chelators, chemicals that attach to and remove iron, can help treat experimental sepsis.[83]

Low-dose aspirin users had a much lower death rate from

bloodstream infection due to the dreaded bacteria *Staphylococcus aureus*, as much as 60% lower compared to non-users.[84] Since invasive microorganisms require a supply of iron, and long-term aspirin use lowers iron, then denying the metal to the invaders could very well be the mechanism that leads to lower death rates in *S. aureus* sepsis.

Since microbial invaders can requisition ferritin for their own use, keeping iron levels in the low normal range may reduce the incidence of infections and/or reduce their severity. Having plenty of iron just lying around waiting for pathogens to use, well, that's asking for trouble.

Multiple sclerosis

Multiple sclerosis (MS) is an autoimmune disease of unknown origin. In it, nerve cells in the brain and spinal cord suffer demyelinization, or damage to their insulating covers. It is progressive and serious; fatigue and weakness are prominent symptoms.

Could iron have something to do with it? The nerve lesions in multiple sclerosis are loaded with iron.[85] In experimental autoimmune encephalitis, which is an animal model used to study MS, 70% of animals with normal or high iron levels got the disease, but none of the animals with iron deficiency did.

An Italian doctor, Paolo Zamboni, believes that obstructed blood flow away from the brain causes iron accumulation leading to MS. Up to 90% of MS patients show signs of blocked cerebral blood flow. He performed an operation on a number of them to unblock the blood flow, and after two years, 73% of his patients no longer had symptoms of MS.[86]

Whether this is the complete story of MS is not known, and most of the medical community doesn't accept that it is. But given that iron is a reactive metal involved in many diseases and in aging, and given Dr. Zamboni's results, it wouldn't be surprising. It looks to be a case of an anatomical abnormality, whether congenital or acquired, that leads to iron overload in the affected areas.

Since removing iron through a relatively simple operation doesn't require a long course of expensive drug treatment, don't expect to hear much about it. It just doesn't generate big profits for doctors or pharmaceutical firms.

Gout

Gout is a form of arthritis that features elevated levels of uric acid, and attacks of gout can be extremely painful, commonly affecting the joint of the big toe. Causes are unknown, though dietary components, especially fructose (from sugar) have been implicated.

In experimental animals, iron can complex with uric acid to form crystals, which are a feature of gout.

A study was undertaken to see whether lowering iron levels in humans with gout had an effect on their disease. The patients received periodic phlebotomy until their iron stores reach "near-iron deficiency", which represents a ferritin level of about 30 ng/ml. At this level, iron stores in the liver are "negligible". After the patients' ferritin levels were lowered, they received periodic phlebotomy to keep them low.[87]

In the two years preceding the trial, total cumulative attacks of gout in these patients were 53 and 48 respectively. In the beginning year of the trial and for two years afterward, the number of attacks was 32, 11, and 7, respectively.

From the year with the greatest number of attacks to the year with the lowest, the number of attacks was reduced by nearly 80%. The chart below shows the results in terms of number of attacks per year for each patient who participated in the trial.

Impressive, no? It certainly looks like iron is one of the factors involved in attacks of gout. Although the author of the study, Dr. Francesco Facchini of Stanford University, stated that it would be "premature" to suggest phlebotomy as a treatment for gout, he wrote that "there is an urgent need to overcome the dogmatic credence that appreciable amounts of iron should always be maintained in storage at any age and by all means."

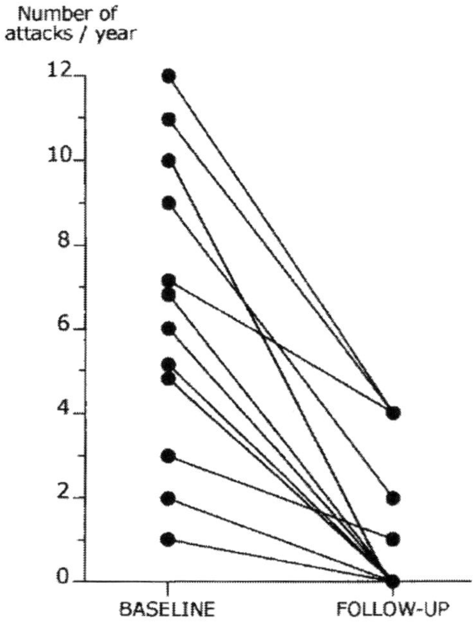
Number of attacks / year
12
10
8
6
4
2
0
BASELINE
FOLLOW-UP

In other words, at least in the case of gout, along with many other conditions, higher levels of stored iron are not necessarily better, and may in fact be much worse. Any other interpretation is outdated dogma.

Chronic Obstructive Pulmonary Disease and Cystic Fibrosis

Chronic obstructive pulmonary disease (COPD) is characterized by poor airflow in and out of the lungs, and the most common symptoms are shortness of breath, sputum production, and chronic cough. Symptoms typically worsen over time. The most common cause of COPD is cigarette smoking, and an estimated 5% of the world's population has it to some degree.

So, if it's caused mainly by smoking cigarettes, how in the world could iron be involved?

It turns out that tobacco is loaded with iron.[88] Someone who smokes one pack of cigarettes a day can inhale about one microgram of iron per day, and macrophages (immune cells) in the lungs of smokers can contain as much as six times the amount of iron as in non-smokers. Iron could be one of the most important toxic compounds in cigarette smoke.

A study using mice found that those animals that lacked a certain protein involved in iron metabolism, IRP2, which is also elevated in the lungs of humans with COPD, were completely protected from damage by cigarette smoke.[89]

Furthermore, mice that were given an iron chelator to remove iron, or mice that were fed a low-iron diet, were also protected from damage to their lungs by cigarette smoke.

The fact that mice were protected from smoke damage by a low-iron diet is particularly important. Because iron in COPD is inside lung cells, it doesn't necessarily follow that less dietary iron will decrease it in lung cells. But in this case, it did.

Whether lowering iron will be of benefit in humans with COPD, or whether it will merely prevent it, as it appears it will, is another question. It's possible that the damage has been done and that lowering iron won't help. On the other hand, if the iron in COPD lung cells generates massive oxidative stress, which it does, then lowering it ought to be of benefit.

I know that if I had COPD I would certainly look into lowering my iron. It's a treatment with a very low risk / benefit ratio, i.e. in most cases there's no harm in trying, and great benefit if successful.

Iron is also involved in the lung disease **cystic fibrosis**, in which most of the pathology involves infection of the lungs with a number of different types of bacteria.[90] High amounts of iron are found in the airways in cystic fibrosis, and disease-causing bacteria require iron for their growth and the ability to invade healthy tissue. What appears to be happening is that excess iron accumulates in the cells lining the airways, which then seeps out into the airway fluids. Bacteria then have all the iron that they need to grow and multiply.

In normal airways, not enough iron is available for invasive bacteria to gain a foothold.

In cystic fibrosis, whole-body iron overload is not the problem; rather, a genetic defect results in excess iron in the airways. This knowledge opens the way for the use of iron chelators to mop up excess iron, remove it from airways, and deny the use of iron to invading pathogens.

Liver Disease

Liver disease can be caused by excessive alcohol consumption, hepatitis viruses, and several other things, such as toxins or obesity. Hemochromatosis, or hereditary iron overload, is one of those other causes. Could iron be involved in other cases of liver disease?

Non-alcoholic fatty liver disease (NAFLD) affects up to 30% of people in the Western world, and is strongly associated with obesity, insulin resistance, and diabetes. Iron in the liver may be elevated in many cases.[91] Phlebotomy, which lowers iron, improves insulin sensitivity in NAFLD, as well as markers of liver damage.[92]

Although the role of iron in NAFLD remains controversial, it's clear that a sizable fraction of patients has iron overload in the liver, and that lowering it may improve their condition. Some researchers have called for more extensive study of phlebotomy for this condition.[93]

Liver disease caused by **hepatitis** can be ameliorated by phlebotomy, and iron is considered a "co-morbid" factor in chronic viral hepatitis.[94]

In a group of patients with viral hepatitis who had phlebotomy such that their iron levels dropped to a very low level (10 ng/ml ferritin) and who were maintained that way for five years, disease progression was much lower.[95]

A group of patients with chronic hepatitis C who received phlebotomy and who were instructed to follow a low-iron diet were followed for a number of years, and were compared to a group who declined iron reduction therapy. After ten years, 39% of the group that had declined iron-reduction therapy had developed liver cancer; only 8.6% of the iron-depletion group developed liver cancer, for a reduction of risk of 43% after adjustment for other factors.[96]

That's a huge risk reduction. It seems clear that iron is highly involved in the progression of chronic liver disease caused by hepatitis C to liver cancer, and that lowering iron via phlebotomy radically reduces the risk.

Chronic ingestion of large amounts of alcohol causes **alcoholic liver disease**. Strange to say, but iron is also involved in this.[97] Alcoholism is associated with increased iron in the liver, and alcohol and iron act synergistically to damage the liver.[98] Alcoholics have greatly increased iron absorption due to the iron-enhancing effect of alcohol, which leads to iron overload.

Iron chelators have been suggested in the treatment of alcoholic liver disease. It seems likely that merely decreasing iron in alcoholics could substantially improve their health. (Although if someone is drinking himself to death, perhaps he doesn't care much about iron. Maybe chelators could be added to booze.)

In laboratory animals, a type of liver failure induced by carbon tetrachloride is widely used as a model of liver failure. In one such experiment, the animals were divided into groups, and one group was treated with n-acetylcysteine (a compound that delivers the amino acid cysteine) and an iron chelator. This group had a survival rate from liver failure of 80%, compared to only 5% in the rats who got neither.[99]

In many or most cases of liver disease, iron is at the very least a co-factor. This can be seen in both animal experiments and in humans, in both of which lowering iron stores prevents or treats liver disease of varying types.

For someone with liver disease, the first step is to eliminate the cause, which may be excessive sugar or carbohydrates in NAFLD, or alcohol in alcoholic liver disease. In viral hepatitis, eliminating the cause may not be possible.

After taking care of the main or putative cause, lowering iron could be the next step. It's what I would do. Patients with liver disease can't donate blood, but natural or synthetic iron chelators, blocking iron absorption from the diet, or if a doctor is willing, therapeutic phlebotomy, are all options.

Frailty and other conditions of aging

As humans age, many of their organs and tissues seemingly wear out or become much less functional with age. Besides the brain, which we covered in a previous chapter, these tissues and organs include the skeletal muscles and bone.

As we get older, we lose muscle, and this starts to occur as early as the decade of the thirties. (See my books **Muscle Up** and **Stop the Clock** for much more on this.) When muscle loss goes on long enough, it becomes **sarcopenia**, or muscle wasting, and it affects every aspect of life. Elderly people with sarcopenia become frail and often dependent on others for help in daily life. They often fall and injure themselves merely because they have difficulty walking or even holding themselves up.

The accumulation of iron in muscle tissue contributes wholly or partially to the genesis of sarcopenia.[100] Iron in muscle damages the mitochondria, the cells' powerhouses, and leads to atrophy and decay of the muscle via oxidative damage. Calorie restriction, which as we saw in a previous chapter hinders the accumulation of iron, also protects against sarcopenia.

In laboratory rats, the accumulation of iron in muscle happens side by side with atrophy (wasting), and calorie restriction protects against iron accumulation.[101] In these same rats, calorie-restricted animals also retained a greater grip strength into an older age than animals that fed freely. Hence it's clear that iron is involved and perhaps required in the pathogenesis of sarcopenia, and that impeding iron accumulation can prevent it.

In a group of Korean women, high ferritin (iron) levels were associated with nearly double the risk of sarcopenia.[102]

Sarcopenia is strongly associated with disuse, and exercise, especially strength training, potently prevents sarcopenia – use it or lose it. One of the biochemical abnormalities associated with muscle disuse is the dysregulation of iron metabolism, allowing iron to "escape" from its normal locked-down status to become free iron, and damage muscle cells.

Preventing or fixing the accumulation of iron may stop muscle wasting.

Osteoporosis

Very high iron load as seen in the condition of

hemochromatosis (hereditary iron overload) or in patients who have received numerous transfusions is a risk factor for **osteoporosis**, the pathological thinning of bones.[103] What we would really like to know is whether iron levels that are high but within the normal range also predispose to osteoporosis.

The issue isn't simple. While older women have up to a 50% rate of osteoporosis, men have a much lower rate, around 20%, and men have higher iron stores than women. But there could be protective factors in men, such as male sex hormones or greater bone mineral density to begin with, or women may have a combination of factors, such as low estrogen combined with increased iron. [104]

Higher iron levels in laboratory animals (rats) causes thinning of bones, and chelating the iron (removing it) makes bones strong.[105]

It's likely that higher iron levels in post-menopausal women play a role in the development of osteoporosis, but more research is needed.

Age-Related Macular Degeneration

Age-related macular degeneration (AMD) is the leading cause of blindness and visual deterioration in the Western world. Oxidative damage to the cells in the retina appears to be the major cause of AMD.

Iron is a potent generator of oxidative damage, and the retinal cells in people with AMD have more iron that in those with normal vision.[106] Smoking greatly raises the risk of AMD, and smoking is known to disrupt iron homeostasis.

Iron chelators have been suggested for treatment of AMD. Controlling high iron levels and/or disruption of iron regulation may help prevent it.

Skin wrinkles

The skin of old people becomes wrinkled, and old people also have higher levels of iron. Is there a connection? Yes – of course!

A group of researchers looked at a group of 12 women, all Caucasian, half of them pre-menopausal, average age 42, half of them post-menopausal, average age 59. They took skin biopsies, and measured ferritin (iron) and antioxidant capacity in the skin.[107]

In the post-menopausal women, ferritin levels were 42% higher than in the pre-menopausal women. Antioxidant capacity was 45% lower in the post-menopausal women. Very straightforward.

After menopause, women no longer lose large amounts of iron through menstrual blood flow. The iron then begins to build up in their bodies until, after a couple decades or so, iron levels begin to approach that of men.

Their rates of heart disease, cancer, and diabetes also rise.

Their skin becomes more wrinkled. Oxidative damage is a prime cause of skin wrinkling. This study shows that the buildup of iron in the women's bodies also includes the skin. Normally, the skin doesn't contain much iron, but a general buildup of iron in the body "spills over" into the skin. Antioxidant capacity in the skin is lower probably precisely because iron is higher. The antioxidant system becomes overwhelmed by highly reactive iron and a state of oxidative stress in the skin comes into being.

Damage including wrinkles results.

Importantly for this study, the measure of iron was ferritin, not free iron. The body strives to keep free iron under control by locking it down in the ferritin molecule, as free iron is a dangerous reactant. In this case, the fact that ferritin went up shows the association between it and free iron: the higher the ferritin, the higher the free iron. They are closely correlated in otherwise healthy people.

The addition of ultraviolet (UV) radiation from the sun to iron-loaded skin causes even more oxidative damage. When UV radiation from the sun hits skin cells, it causes degradation of the safe-storage ferritin molecule and the release of free iron, causing oxidative damage to the skin; in fact, this is probably the main way that the sun inflicts damage to skin.[108] Iron chelators – chemicals that remove iron from the body – actually protect cells from solar radiation damage.[109]

Release of iron in the skin after sun exposure could also be a prime mechanism in the development of skin cancer.

Since solar radiation causes the release of free iron from ferritin, then the best way to ensure against skin damage from the sun is to have low ferritin in the first place so less free iron is released. So in the case of wrinkled or damaged skin, the same methods for lowering iron that prevent or treat other conditions work here.

Topical iron chelators, which remove iron from the skin, may be useful in combating wrinkles, although keeping body iron levels from becoming elevated and thus preventing wrinkles in the first place is a better strategy. Whether lowering iron in the skin either directly with topical chelators or indirectly by whole-body lowering would help already wrinkled skin isn't known just now, but I would certainly give it a try.

Kojic acid is a naturally derived agent that is used in skin-lightening soaps and lotions, and it reportedly actually works. It also chelates iron, removing it from the skin, and this may have a lot to do with its effects. Whether it also removes wrinkles - well, give it a shot and report back.

Oral contraceptives

Oral contraceptives – birth control pills – are associated

with higher risks of thrombosis (blood clots), cancer, and heart attack. For instance, studies have found as much as a 3.5-fold increase in the risk of thrombosis.[110] A 50% increase in the rate of breast cancer has been found in long-term oral contraceptive users.[111]

Oral contraceptives greatly decrease the amount of a woman's menstrual blood flow, in some cases cutting it nearly in half.[112] This leads to much higher iron levels in women who use them.[113]

Is increased iron behind the increased health risks of birth control pills? That wouldn't be surprising, yet no one ever discusses the possibility. Why no discussion?

As stated before, scientists and doctors become very enamored of their theories and can be reluctant to give them up, even in the face of compelling evidence. In this case, iron is such a simple story that it would invalidate years of research.

Birth Defects

Could iron cause birth defects?

Weeks 3 to 8 of human pregnancy make up the embryonic period. During this time, the mother absorbs 30% less iron than needed, suggesting a mechanism to limit iron. Iron also strongly promotes morning sickness, which suggests that the mother and fetus are trying to get rid of it.[114]

In mice during early pregnancy, iron causes birth defects.

All of this is merely suggestive, but the author of the cited article argues that pregnant women should be tested for ferritin and not supplemented if the level is high enough, and that if needed, supplementation should wait until after week 8 of pregnancy.

Grey Hair

Aging is obviously associated with gray hair, and iron might be connected to it, since iron increases in aging. Grey hair seems to be caused by oxidative stress in the hair follicle, causing loss of detoxifying enzymes, as a result of which the hair becomes effectively bleached.

In young men with prematurely greying hair, iron levels were higher.[115] Sadly, very little research seems to have been done on this.

Iron and Animals: Is Commercial Pet Food Killing Your Pets?

In the course of my research on iron, aging, and disease, I interviewed Dr. Eugene D. Weinberg, emeritus professor of biology at Indiana University, whose life work concerns the biological actions of iron, on which he's published more than 140 scientific papers. He kindly wrote a preface to this book.

Dr. Weinberg mentioned to me, totally in passing, that many commercial pet foods contain seriously high amounts of iron. I'm sure hardly anyone else in the world knows this, and if anyone knows, that person would be Dr. Weinberg.

I set out to verify the facts behind his assertion. Information on the amount of iron in commercial pet foods is very difficult to find.

However, in the course of reading a scientific paper on iron metabolism, I came across the statement that, while laboratory mice are estimated to have an iron requirement of 35 ppm (parts per million) of their diet, some laboratory mouse chow contains 10 times that amount.[116] This is an astonishing statement, because if scientists experiment with mice, and feed them toxic levels of iron, that might invalidate many of their results.

LabDiet, "the world leader in laboratory animal nutrition", has a mouse diet, and the company provides a detailed analysis of its content.[117] Iron is listed at 200 ppm. In this case, that's about 6 times the requirement of mice – not 10 times, but close enough – which is still more than enough to cause iron overload in animals that eat it.

The iron requirement for both cats and dogs has been estimated at 80 ppm.[118] LabDiet also makes a feline diet, and their analysis states that it contains 290 ppm, or about 3.6 times the requirement.[119] As an animal ages, this amount of iron will produce iron overloading. Well, I suppose lab cats aren't destined to live long anyway, poor animals.

If LabDiet, a company which presumably takes great pains to ensure proper nutrition in animals, loads their mouse and cat diets with iron, do commercial pet food companies load dog and cat food with iron also?

Unfortunately, I was unable to find an analysis as detailed as the mouse diet for dog and cat food. (Maybe they don't want you to know; one major pet food company did not return my calls and emails.) But I did find that most of them have been fortified with iron. Purina Dog Chow is fortified with ferrous sulfate, a form of iron, and Blue Buffalo dog food is fortified with iron amino acid chelate, another form. AAFCO, a consortium of government officials involved in animal feed, previously stated that a maximum of 3000 ppm iron was acceptable in dog food, but this statement was rescinded, and now any maximum amount is apparently acceptable.[120] Note that this is 37.5 times the iron requirement of dogs.

Now, humans shouldn't take iron supplements unless there's a demonstrated need and a doctor advises it. Yet our pets are eating iron-supplemented food all the time, though how much iron they get and how iron-overloaded they become isn't known at this point – but it seems to be a lot.

Iron overload due to pet food loaded with toxic amounts of iron could be killing pets or making them die before their time. That's not only possible, but in my opinion probable.

How long are dogs and cats supposed to live?

The natural lifespan of a cat is allegedly about 15 years, but perhaps that figure is skewed downward by bad food. In other words, maybe 15 years is the "unnatural" lifespan caused by eating toxic amounts of iron in commercial pet food.

Consider the case of Creme Puff, the world's longest lived cat, who lived to the age of 38, well beyond the age most cats live.[121] When most people learn about Creme Puff, they figure, like I did, that her long life must have been some kind of fluke, perhaps genetic. But then one learns that the same man who owned Creme Puff also owned another, unrelated cat, Grandpa, who lived to the age of 34. Clearly, this man must have been doing something right for his cats. Two very long-lived and unrelated cats in the same household doesn't look like a fluke, but must be related to their environment.

One thing their owner did right was that he didn't feed them commercial pet food. He fed them bacon and eggs, coffee and cream, and vegetables. His cats didn't become iron-loaded from commercial pet food – at least I think that's a likely possibility for the long life of his cats.

Pets have been getting fatter at the same time that humans

have. Many have blamed the carbohydrates in commercial pet food for pet obesity, and that may very well be a contributor, but iron could play a role there too. Cats often get diabetes and kidney failure, both conditions that are associated with iron overload (among other things). Dogs get cancer, in which iron is also a factor.

Whether iron overload is a major problem for dogs and cats is necessarily speculative, as it appears that hardly anyone has looked into this issue. Just as with humans, the dangers of iron are largely overlooked or unappreciated. I think it is a distinct possibility, and that without iron-loaded commercial pet food, dogs and cats might live considerably longer and healthier than they do now. I've already stopped feeding commercial cat food to my cat.

Takeaway points

- Iron is involved in many other diseases, including infections, multiple sclerosis, gout, liver disease, cystic fibrosis, COPD, and macular degeneration
- Iron may be the mechanism behind health risks of birth control pills
- Iron might cause birth defects
- Iron damages skin and may cause gray hair

- Iron-fortified pet food could be causing iron overload and early death in cats and dogs

7: How to take control of your iron and your health

A few easy steps to better health

The evidence set forth in this book shows that avoiding excess iron in the body is not only a worthwhile thing to do for health, but is crucial.

Lower iron (but not iron deficiency) means less cancer, heart disease, diabetes, frailty, and brain disorders. Inhibition of iron increases lifespan in lab animals, and ought to do so in humans.

I had my own ferritin measured not long ago. It was 137, a level I consider too high and that puts my health at risk. I already have most of my health risks covered: I exercise, eat right, and stay lean. But having a high iron (ferritin) could offset the health benefits of diet and exercise, and if high enough, could negate them entirely.

Furthermore, preventing or fixing excess iron is not terribly difficult. A few easy steps and you could be on your way to much better health.

Doctors and most mainstream health advice will not tell you about the dangers of excess iron, because they don't know about it, and they care even less. On top of that, doctors routinely prescribe iron supplements to their patients even without demonstrated iron deficiency. Many people – about 15% of adults – take them on their own because they believe it's a healthy thing to do.

Doctors do know all about hemochromatosis, or hereditary iron overload, as this is a well-known condition that, if untreated, can result in cancer, liver disease, and early death. But in hemochromatosis, iron levels are sky high, much higher than the levels that we've been discussing in this book for their ability to cause disease. Hemochromatosis is hard to overlook, given some straightforward lab tests and a physical examination.

If you see your doctor and for one reason or another get your iron level tested, unless the result is clearly abnormally high, your doctor will very likely not believe that it's a problem and will take no action.

With that in mind, let's take a look at what a normal, that is, healthy, iron level is, and at what level of increase it starts to cause health problems.

Normal iron: what it is and isn't

The most common laboratory test for iron is the ferritin test, and from here on, I will be using this term as a synonym for body iron stores. (It's slightly more complicated than that, but is perfectly acceptable for our purposes.)

Ferritin is a protein that the body uses to sequester iron. Since iron is a reactive metal, the body strives to keep iron well under control by forming a complex of it with other molecules, and ferritin is the most important iron storage molecule.

Hemoglobin, however, contains most of the body's iron, around 80% of it. Hemoglobin is the molecule used by red blood cells to carry oxygen to the body, and iron is necessary for this function. The most important consequence of iron deficiency is an insufficient amount of hemoglobin, and as a consequence the blood doesn't function optimally.

Iron is also used in other crucial functions, such as energy generation and detoxification.

When the need for iron by hemoglobin and other molecules and functions is satisfied, and more iron is ingested, it is stored as ferritin. Thus, a hemoglobin level in a normal, healthy person has an upper limit, but ferritin can rise without limit.

Normal laboratory values

If your doctor orders a ferritin test – or you get him or her to order it for you – the result will be accompanied by a so-called "normal range", also called a reference range or normal laboratory values. The normal range is calculated such that 95% of apparently healthy people have a value within that range.

For ferritin, the Mayo Clinic states that a typical reference range is 11 to 307 ng/ml for women, and 24 to 336 for men. If a ferritin value is lower than the lower limit of the reference range, a patient may be iron deficient, and above that may have iron overload. A number within the reference range is deemed normal.

Absent clear signs and symptoms of deficiency or overload, a doctor is unlikely to take any action if a ferritin test value falls within the normal range. In fact, most doctors are unlikely to take even a second glance at *any* test whose value is not clearly abnormal.

But since iron is an under-recognized factor in disease risk, as I've argued in this book, many people whose ferritin value falls within the normal range have, in reality, a value that is too high.

Besides ferritin, there is no other lab test that I'm aware of whose normal value spans more than a ten-fold range from low to high. The Mayo Clinic reference range cited above spans a 14-fold range for men, and nearly 28-fold for women. The reference ranges of most lab tests span far less, depending on the particular test, for example a range of 1.5 (potassium) to 3.0 (creatinine) from low to high.

Normal lab values for any substance of interest, including ferritin, are, as mentioned, calculated from the values that 95% of apparently healthy people have. But two thirds of the population are overweight or obese, many have unrecognized blood sugar or other metabolic problems, and most don't exercise or care about what they eat; in short, *laboratory normal values are calculated using the values of unhealthy people.* Many of the apparently healthy people whose test results are within the normal range are at great risk of cancer and heart disease and many other diseases. If you are careful about your health, you need to do a lot better than the lab normal range, and find out what the *optimal* values are.

The conclusion is that the normal ranges are not normal. Disease risk from iron begins, depending on the disease, at levels *within the normal range.* Therefore, *for optimal health, you must disregard the normal range.*

The optimal level of iron

Based on the considerations above, suppose you're an adult man, get a ferritin test, and the result is 200 ng/ml, which is a not uncommon number and within the normal range. You ask your doctor about it, and he or she says that there is no cause for concern. Should you be concerned? What is an optimal level of ferritin anyway?

A large body of evidence shows that health benefits accrue by lowering ferritin starting from the upper limits of the reference range down to just above the minimum needed to prevent iron deficiency.[122]

A study in Korea found that men in the highest quartile (fourth) of ferritin levels had nearly double the risk of developing type 2 diabetes as men in the lowest. The upper quartile represented a ferritin of 284 or higher. Importantly, risk of diabetes increased from the lowest level, that is, risk rose as ferritin rose.[123] All within the normal range.

A meta-analysis of five studies found that, for women, risk of diabetes increased at threshold ferritin levels of between 86 and 150, and for men, between 184 and 300.[124] Note that all of these values are within the normal range.

Men who had ferritin levels greater than 300 were nearly *five times more likely* to be diagnosed with diabetes. For women, having a ferritin greater than 150 increased the likelihood of a diabetes diagnosis 3.6 times.[125] All within the normal range.

In men, increased risk of having coronary artery calcification was seen at a ferritin greater than 257. This is within the normal range. (Tired of reading that yet?)

In women, ferritin greater than 137 was associated with increased risk of stroke.[126]

In healthy men, increased ferritin meant more oxidative stress and insulin resistance. An important point about this study is that, not only were these markers of worse health seen in men with normal ferritin values, but that they increased continuously from the lowest third (<97) to the highest (>180).

One piece of evidence shows that reducing iron stores down to a very low level has benefits compared to those who already have a low ferritin. This evidence concerns blood vessel function, in particular something called flow-mediated dilation. The decline in this function is closely linked to atherosclerosis, the hardening of the arteries, and high flow-mediated dilation means that blood vessels are in a more youthful and healthy state. Two groups of blood donors were compared: 1) high-frequency donors, who had donated at least eight times in the previous two years; and 2) low-frequency donors, who had donated no more than once in each of the previous two years. (Note that this method of comparison eliminates the healthy donor effect.) The high-frequency donors had an average serum ferritin level of 17, which is quite low, and the low-frequency donors an average of 52, still quite low when compared to population averages. Flow-mediated dilation in high-frequency donors was much better than in low-frequency, about 44% better.[127]

The point is clear: iron overload that has adverse health effects begins at a much lower level than most doctors believe, a level within the "normal" range.

The reader might also wonder that since the studies I've cited reveal only associations, they don't show cause and effect. Maybe it's just a coincidence that higher levels of ferritin are associated with worse health, which is caused by something else and only coincidentally raises iron in the body.

In opposition to the idea that it's all just a coincidence, a number of studies show improved health or lower risk of disease when iron is lowered. Some of these have already been discussed previously, for instance, cancer risk was 40% lower and death from cancer 60% lower in men who underwent phlebotomy (bloodletting) to lower their iron, as opposed to men who did not.[128]

Reducing ferritin through phlebotomy lowers insulin resistance, an important marker of ill health.[129] The same subjects had increased HDL cholesterol, lower triglycerides, lower blood pressure, which represent improvements in cardiovascular disease risk.

It is not all just a coincidence. Ferritin levels that are capable of harming health can fall within the normal range.

What remains to be determined is the optimal level of ferritin. The answer to this question is necessarily somewhat speculative, but we can arrive at a decent estimate.

Low iron and iron deficiency

It's worth reiterating that iron is a required nutrient and that it's possible to become deficient in it, which can lead to anemia, fatigue, and other health problems.

Iron deficiency should be avoided. At what level of ferritin does a human become deficient?

In contrast to excess iron, the normal ranges for ferritin are actually a decent guide in the matter of iron deficiency. Historically, iron deficiency has been a much bigger problem than iron overload, so it's been studied extensively and doctors are very aware of it.

Therefore, a ferritin level of less than 20 should be avoided. Since this is not an absolute number applicable to everyone, staying above that value by perhaps 10 points may be a good idea.

Many of the studies on phlebotomy to lower iron levels used periodic blood withdrawal, calibrated to the individual patient, to drop ferritin levels to "near iron deficiency", a level just above that which would cause deficiency. For instance, in the study on insulin sensitivity, after the course of periodic phlebotomy, the subjects average ferritin level was 13, which is very low indeed.

The benefits of lower ferritin increase all the way down until iron deficiency develops. Barring deficiency, it appears that the lower, the better.

A review of this issue concluded that optimum adult ferritin values are in the range of 20 to 40 for women, and 50 to 70 for men. Within these ranges, both iron deficiency and iron overload can be avoided.[130]

These ranges are narrow, much more so than actual "normal ranges" that clinical laboratories use. In particular, the upper limit is much lower.

How to control your iron level

Lowering your iron stores, or preventing the rise of high iron in the first place, can be done a number of ways.

As iron is necessary for growth and development, lowering iron stores is not for children, adolescents, and pregnant women. Fertile (that is, pre-menopausal) women, while they may benefit from it, are unlikely to need to lower iron, as blood loss from the menstrual cycle keeps iron naturally low. As we've seen, the average ferritin level of a fertile woman is around 35 ng/ml, and this is a safe level that does not promote disease or aging.

In men, iron levels start to rise at about the age of 19, and by the decade of their thirties they usually have far more iron than women the same age. In women, iron starts rising after menopause (or hysterectomy), and slowly rises toward that of men, although on average they never catch up.

Iron stores (ferritin levels) rise slowly. In the case of adult men, from maturity to the decade of their thirties, ferritin increases on average about 100 points, so the annual increase is on the order of 5 to 10 points. Absent blood donation, they decrease slowly too, so if you attempt a low-iron diet and feel a bit off shortly after, it's not from lack of iron.

Adult men and post-menopausal women are those most likely to benefit from decreasing their iron stores.

Before undertaking any intervention to lower iron, you should know your ferritin and hemoglobin numbers. Both of these are common lab tests performed by almost all clinical labs, but they require a doctor's orders. Hemoglobin is a part of a test panel known as a CBC (complete blood count), and doctors often order a CBC on patients as part of an annual physical or checkup. In addition, they often order a CBC test panel on any patient that has any illness other than a minor one. So, lots of people reading this may well already have a CBC test report on file; if you've had lab tests recently, you can ask your doctor for a copy of your CBC, assuming you've had one.

Doctors do not routinely order ferritin tests, usually doing so only in cases of suspected iron deficiency or overload, or to rule out these conditions, so you may have to ask for one.

If you have a high ferritin and are making a concerted effort to lower it, and you want to periodically test for ferritin, you should ask your doctor for a standing order to get tested. That way you can get tested when you like, and don't need to contact the doctor every time you want a test. In iron overload clinics, a typical standing order may be for four tests a year. Of course, you need not use all the tests in your standing order, but they'll be available if and when you want them.

You can go another route for your ferritin testing: The Life Extension Foundation offers a ferritin test for, at last check, $28.

If you don't know your ferritin and hemoglobin numbers, you can still use some of the techniques below to lower your iron.

However, if your ferritin is very high, say from 300 to over 1000, you will need a concerted effort to get your iron down to a low, safe level. If you don't know that number, you won't have any idea of how much you should do in the way of iron-lowering interventions. So you want to know. You shouldn't, after reading this book, just consider drinking some tea with your meals or taking a supplement or two and think that all will be well. If your iron is very high, all will not be well.

If after getting your ferritin tested and it's over 300, you should periodically get retested to monitor your iron level and see how well your iron-lowering interventions are working. If it is that high, your doctor may be interested in working with you to lower it.

If your ferritin level is low, in the range we discussed (20 to 40 for women, 50 to 70 for men), then practicing any of the interventions discussed below could put you at risk for iron deficiency, so that's another reason to know your iron level.

However, the risk of iron deficiency is low even if you have a low normal ferritin because, if low iron leads to low hemoglobin (anemia), you will not be eligible to donate blood, which eliminates the major means of lowering iron. When it comes to donating blood, there's a feedback loop: if your hemoglobin, and thus iron, drops too low, you can't donate.

There are four ways to lower iron levels or to prevent iron accumulation:

- Blood donation
- Iron chelation
- Inhibition of iron absorption from food
- Low-iron diet

Blood donation

Donating blood at the Red Cross or other blood banks is the surest, most effective, and fastest method of lowering iron.

Whole blood or red cell donations are the only types that lower iron, as most iron is found in red blood cells, not plasma or platelets. Plasma or platelet donations have little to no effect in lowering iron.

When someone volunteers to donate blood, the blood bank measures the donor's hemoglobin level during the screening process, and if the hemoglobin level is too low, donation will not be allowed. They do this for the donor's safety, since a blood donation also decreases hemoglobin, and if the donor's hemoglobin is already low, then it could decrease to a low, potentially unhealthy and unsafe level.

Low hemoglobin can be caused by a number of things, one of the most common being iron deficiency. So on the bright side, if your hemoglobin is too low to donate, your iron likely doesn't need to be lowered anyway.

If hemoglobin is within the normal range (which differs between men and women, men having higher hemoglobin), and all other screening factors give the go-ahead signal, then donation proceeds.

Hemoglobin is not iron

Blood bank personnel often have a habit of referring to a donor's hemoglobin number as their iron level. It is not. Hemoglobin is hemoglobin, not ferritin or some other form of iron.

Don't confuse hemoglobin with iron. If the blood bank nurse tells you that your iron is 15 (or some other similar number), that's normal, but does not represent your iron level. A normal hemoglobin is completely compatible with an abnormally high iron level, hence it's important to keep the distinction clear.

Why they do that I don't know; perhaps they don't want to confuse people, or perhaps they're a little confused themselves.

Blood banks do not measure ferritin or any other iron level when you donate. They measure hemoglobin, or sometimes hematocrit, another measure of blood that is also not iron.

Whole blood and double red cell donations

A whole-blood donation consists of the removal of about 450 milliliters of blood in the U.S., but in some other countries may be 500 ml. Since the average adult human has a blood volume of about 5 liters, a blood donation removes about 10% of one person's total blood supply.

Red blood cells, which hold the iron-containing hemoglobin, generally make up about 40 to 50% of the total blood volume in men, and from 35 to 45% in women. This number is known as the hematocrit, a test which is part of a complete blood count. The remaining blood volume is the liquid portion, known as plasma.

A red cell donation is similar to a whole-blood donation, but in this case only red blood cells are removed via a machine, and plasma is returned to the donor. Red cell donations sometimes come in the form of "double red cell" donations, in which you donate twice the amount of red blood cells as a whole blood donation.

Double red cell donations have the advantage that you rid yourself of iron twice as much with only one donation. They have the disadvantage that they're going to leave you a little fatigued and with lower exercise capacity for longer.

Double red cell donations may be spontaneously offered to a donor, especially if he's a large, healthy man, or you may need to ask for one if you're interested.

Since the total body iron content of an adult man is 3 to 4 grams, and blood contains about 80% of this iron, one whole-blood donation removes roughly 250 mg of iron, depending on the individual. Even a person with a high iron load loses about the same amount, since high iron is a matter of high ferritin, not hemoglobin, and hemoglobin (in red blood cells) is what's being removed.

After a donation, blood volume recovers fairly quickly, probably in a matter of hours, and less than 24 hours. The Red Cross recommends that donors do no heavy exercise nor drink alcohol on the day of the donation, since a lower blood volume could make these activities less safe, given a lower blood volume. Other activities, such as office or house work, are fine.

The loss of red blood cells takes longer to recover from than blood volume. Blood donors must wait a minimum of two months between donations; by this time, red blood cells are fully replenished, although in healthy people with adequate nutrition, the replenishment time is likely much shorter than that.

To replenish red blood cells, the body must make more hemoglobin to put inside those cells. Since iron is required for hemoglobin, the body takes iron from storage, mostly ferritin, and uses it to make hemoglobin. Hence, blood donation lowers iron. For a blood donor, the ferritin value doesn't decline immediately upon donation, but declines as new red cells are made in the time after the donation. A ferritin test done within two months after a blood donation therefore captures a declining value; to get an accurate picture of your body iron stores, ferritin should be tested more than two months after a donation, or at any time before one.

Quantifying the effect of blood donation on iron

While a blood donation lowers body iron stores by about 250 mg, we're more interested in its effect on ferritin, since that's the most common measure of iron stores.

A rule of thumb is that one whole-blood donation lowers

ferritin by about 30 ng/ml, though some observers say it is up to 50.

Hence if your ferritin was 120 before a donation, around one to two months after it, it would be about 70 to 90.

If multiple donations are made, say several in a year, a couple of different things occur. One is that ferritin levels drop further with more donations; the second is that the body responds to a drop in ferritin by activating hormones that increase iron uptake from food. This makes sense, as the body senses a drop in iron and the need for more, and therefore it ramps up iron intake.

Essentially, with more donations, in terms of lowering iron, you have to run faster to stay in the same place. This doesn't mean there's any problem in lowering ferritin to a low normal range, as we'll see, but lowering it to ultra-low levels and keeping it there may require relatively frequent donations.

To get a handle on how much in the way of blood donation is required to lower iron, look at the following chart from a Danish study on ferritin values in donors, by frequency of donation, and non-donors.

Table 1. Danish study of the influence of blood donation of serum ferritin levels (ng/mL) in men, 30-66 years of age.[51]

Donation History Per Year	Ferritin Median 5-95 pct*	Ferritin Range
0	137	46-396
2	44	17-122
3	38	14-110
4	31	12-91

* 5th to 95th percentile

The donors were all men, age 30 to 66, and non-donors had an average ferritin of 137, about the same average seen in the U.S. for adult men.

It can be seen that two donations annually dropped ferritin levels dramatically, while the further drop produced by more than two donations was less dramatic.

We don't know for how long the men had been donating blood, and previous, recent donations, say in the year or two prior to the study, would also contribute to lower ferritin. But even at the two donations a year level, the ferritin was solidly within the low normal range that we're striving for.

A study done in the 1970s found that first-time male blood donors, average age in their 30s, had a ferritin of about 127; for females the ferritin was 46. These figures closely track the numbers from other studies concerning average ferritin values in the population. For male donors, one blood donation a year was enough to cut the average ferritin in half. For females, the result was similar though not as strong, which is to be expected since they had lower iron levels to begin with.[131] Based on this study, for a man with an average ferritin, one blood donation annually may be enough to attain and keep a healthy ferritin level.

Now, we also know that the average fertile woman has a ferritin level of about 35. The average fertile woman also loses approximately 35 to 60 ml of blood in her menstrual cycle, or about 420 to 720 ml a year. The first number, 420 ml, is remarkably close to the amount of blood lost in one blood donation, which is 450 ml. The second number is somewhat less than the amount of blood lost in two donations.

Therefore, it follows that, assuming that someone has a relatively normal ferritin to begin with, one blood donation a year may be enough to get it into the low normal range, while two per year would be likely to ensure it.

The number of blood donations required in getting to that low ferritin value in the first place will vary greatly between individuals. For example, if a man has a ferritin of 300, which is not uncommon, and one donation lowers ferritin by 30 points, then getting to a level of 70 may require up to 7 or more donations. While this looks like a lot, someone who's dedicated to lowering a high ferritin can accomplish this in 14 months, with one donation every two months. If we use the figure of 50 for the decrease in ferritin with each donation, then if that man with a 300 ferritin donated blood four times, he would get below 100, and five times would put him squarely in the low normal range.

I know of an 89-year-old woman who started donating blood at the age of 50, and who has given blood 110 times – so far. That's about 3 donations each and every year. The world record for blood donations is held by a Florida man, age 78, who's given whole blood 315 times, amounting to almost 40 gallons of blood. It took him 60 years to accomplish this feat.[132] In the photo accompanying the article about him, he looks fantastically fit and healthy too – is donating blood the secret to his good health and youthful appearance? I wouldn't be surprised.

However, if you don't feel quite so zealous about blood donation, one donation a year should be adequate once you've reached the low normal range. This is why you should know your ferritin first, since that gives you an indication of how many donations you'll need to lower your iron.

The Red Cross estimates that only about 38% of the American public are eligible to donate blood, since age, health, and travel history exclude many. Of these, only about 5% actually donate. In case of ineligibility, there are other options for lowering or preventing high iron.

Therapeutic phlebotomy is the withdrawal of blood from the body, and works just like blood donation. The main differences between the two are that therapeutic phlebotomy is a medical procedure specifically designed to lower iron, and the blood is discarded rather than donated. In cases of serious iron overload, patients may undergo one as often as once a week.

Therapeutic phlebotomy is normally designated only for those whose medical conditions indicate it, for example hemochromatosis, or hereditary iron overload. Whether a doctor would prescribe it for lowering iron when it is not grossly overloaded isn't clear, but if one were unable to donate blood, it may be worthwhile asking a doctor if this is an option.

Summary of Blood Donation

1. Each whole blood donation can be expected to lower ferritin by between 30 and 50 points (ng/ml).

2. On average, men who donated once a year cut ferritin values in half. This assumes starting from average, at a ferritin of about 130.

3. Two blood donations a year almost ensures a low normal ferritin, again, starting from an average level.

4. Therefore, to use blood donation to lower ferritin levels, one to two donations a year should do the job,

assuming you start from an average level.

Iron Chelators

Chelators are chemicals, either natural or synthetic, that attach to iron, after which the chelators and the iron are excreted from the body.

A number of synthetic iron chelators are available by prescription. However, some can have fairly serious side effects, some require intravenous administration, and doctors normally prescribe them for serious cases of iron overload only. Therefore, for our purposes, they are not under consideration here.

A number of natural substances that are known for beneficial health effects also chelate iron, which is probably the main reason that they're healthy in the first place. These substances include:

- quercetin
- curcumin
- inositol hexaphosphate (IP6)
- EGCG (from green tea)
- theaflavin (from black tea)

All of these are available as relatively inexpensive, over-the-counter supplements.

Quercetin, a flavonoid found in a number of fruits and vegetables, possesses potent iron-chelating activity, and is known to have the ability to cross the blood-brain barrier.[133] To get the potent chelating activity of quercetin, it's necessary to take it in amounts found in supplements, since the amounts in food are small.

Curcumin, which is the active compound found in the spice turmeric, has been found to induce iron deficiency in mice if given long enough.[134] Again, it must be taken at supplement-level strengths to get the benefit.

Inositol hexaphosphate, commonly known as IP6, is a constituent of vegetables and grains, and pure IP6 as a supplement is derived from rice bran. It has been shown to protect neurons, and has been suggested as a treatment for Parkinson's disease.[135] It also has anticancer effects against numerous different types of cancer cells, virtually every cancer cell that's been tested, undoubtedly connected to its iron-chelating property. It's very cheap if you buy it as a bulk powder. I take IP6 daily, at 500 mg each morning.

EGCG from green tea, and theaflavins from black tea, are, while available as supplements, perhaps more interesting for the fact that tea contains them, which is important in inhibiting iron absorption from food, as we'll see below. EGCG has been shown to be as potent an iron chelator as the prescription iron-chelating drug desferrioxamine; in addition, it can cross into the brain, and for both these reasons has been suggested as a treatment for Alzheimer's disease.[136] We saw above that green tea extract potently prevents prostate cancer in men with a high risk for it, and this is very likely related to its iron-chelating ability.

Getting good results

Most or all of these natural compounds have not undergone clinical trials in humans to determine how well and how much they can remove iron from the body, and their ability to do so is based on experiments using lab animals or cell culture. So there's no hard data on how well they work in people. There are anecdotal reports of people greatly lowering their ferritin levels with some of these compounds, but they are after all just individual stories, so results may vary a lot between different people, depending on dose and lots of other factors.

If you use any of these natural compounds for lowering iron, you should therefore monitor your iron levels using periodic ferritin testing to ensure that you get the results you want.

Clinical trials using these iron chelators are not likely to happen any time soon, since they are all cheap and not patented, and therefore are unable to make profits for pharmaceutical companies. Add to that the fact of a prejudice in favor of drugs for any treatment, along with the generally unrecognized dangers of iron; basically no one in any position to do something about it cares about these natural compounds.

Dosages of these compounds for iron chelation are not known with certainty, and the suggested doses on the label should not be exceeded.

Iron supplements

Perhaps needless to say, if you want to lower iron levels, do not take any iron supplements. Iron supplementation is a common practice, whether under a doctor's advice or not.

I can't tell you how many times I've heard that someone I know takes iron supplements. The vast majority of the time they are doing so without a doctor's advice, and most of them are women.

Fertile women have a higher requirement for iron, but in most cases, it can be met through the diet. Post-menopausal women *do not* have a higher requirement, and their common practice of taking iron supplements harms their health.

Iron supplements should only be taken under a doctor's advice, regardless of your age and sex. Even then, make sure you understand why you are taking them. If you're not actually anemic (with low hemoglobin or microcytic red blood cells), and they're prescribed for some nebulous reason, caution is in order.

Some medical experts believe that much of the iron overload seen in the older population comes from the common practice of taking iron supplements. Many people inadvertently or unknowingly take iron supplements by taking multivitamins that contain iron, as most of them do.

So-called "mature" multivitamins are often formulated without iron, so these would be a better option if you want to take a multivitamin. But be aware that many mature multivitamins also contain copper, and people who take copper supplements also have a higher death rate. Multivitamins almost always contain calcium too, another mineral it would be wise to avoid. Basically, I would just forego a multivitamin altogether.

A recent study found that taking iron supplements could result in acute damage to blood vessels. When exposed to low iron concentrations, cells from blood vessels show immediate DNA damage. These low concentrations of iron are within the range of what could be expected from taking a single iron supplement tablet.[137]

Aspirin

Aspirin is a very interesting drug when it comes to iron reduction.

Aspirin taken at a daily low dose of 80 milligrams – a so-called baby aspirin – has been shown to cause or to be associated with a striking reduction in cancer incidence: a 40 to 50% reduction in colon cancer, an up to 75% reduction in esophageal cancer, and for all cancers, a 25% reduction.[138] The reduction in death from cancer was 37%. The reduction in risk occurs only after three years of taking aspirin, and a greater reduction is seen after five years.

How does aspirin lower cancer risk so dramatically? The most plausible mechanism, in this writer's opinion and in the opinions of a number of other observers, is because it lowers body iron stores.

Cancers have a voracious appetite for iron, since they are fast-growing and iron is required for growth. They over-express certain genes that allow them to grab on to more iron. Iron enhances tumor growth, and iron-deficient mice have less tumor growth. If aspirin lowers iron stores in the body, this provides a solid mechanism for understanding its role in cancer prevention.

People who take aspirin do have lower iron stores, as measured by ferritin, as much as 25% lower for people who take more than 7 regular strength aspirin a week.[139] Low-dose aspirin also results in lower ferritin.

There are at least three plausible ways in which aspirin lowers iron.

1. It chelates iron. In fact, chemists measure the amount of aspirin in a solution by adding iron to make an

aspirin-iron complex, which turns blue and can be measured in a spectrophotometer.

2. It causes synthesis of the protein ferritin molecule, which then captures more iron. In this way, free iron, the most destructive kind, is reduced.

3. It causes bleeding, which lowers iron. Most observers see this as the major mechanism of aspirin's effects on iron.

Aspirin raises the amount of minor intestinal bleeding, which is usually not noticed by the person taking aspirin. If it raised the rate of bleeding by 1 ml (about 20 drops) a day, then these cumulative losses are well within the range of normal menstrual blood loss. Since we know that fertile women have both lower iron and lower rates of disease, this shows how aspirin could be effective at lowering iron, enough so to lower cancer risk.

Unfortunately, aspirin also carries a risk of major bleeding, which is a medical emergency. The risk of major bleeding for users of low-dose aspirin, at less than 300 mg a day, rises about 50%.[140] The absolute rate of major bleeding among aspirin users was 5.6 per 1000 person-years of aspirin use, in contrast to 3.60 for non-users of aspirin.

As seen in the absolute rates of major bleeding, the risk is still relatively low, and even non-users of aspirin have some risk. In addition, risk of bleeding decreased after three years of taking it. But the risk is there.

The risk to benefit ratio of aspirin depends on several things, such as your risk of cancer, risk of bleeding, of heart attack, and so on. While cancer is the number two killer in the U.S., major bleeding is not even in the top ten. Since aspirin decreases risk of both cancer and heart attack (the latter at least in people who have already had one) but raises the risk of bleeding, much depends on a person's age and health status. In someone under the age of perhaps 50 or so, risks may very well outweigh benefits, but benefits may well outweigh risks in older people. Some observers believe that aspirin may be one of the most effective anti-aging drugs currently available.

An online benefit-harm calculator, developed by scientists at the University of Zurich, purports to calculate for anyone, given age, sex, previous health conditions, and risk of heart attack, whether taking low-dose aspirin offers more benefits or more risk of harm. It can be found at benefit-harm-balance.com.

Anyone who wants to take low-dose aspirin should talk to a doctor about the risks versus benefits of doing so. Peter Rothwell, the doctor who has led many of the studies on aspirin use and lower cancer risk, has said, "In terms of prevention, anyone with a family history [of cancer] would be sensible to take aspirin." Other knowledgeable observers have been more cautious, saying that further study is needed.[141]

More studies are unlikely, however, since aspirin is a cheap, generic drug, and no pharmaceutical company can make large profits from it. Most physicians remain reluctant to prescribe aspirin to healthy people.

Inhibition of iron absorption from food

In the modern Western world, iron is difficult to avoid. We eat quite a bit of red meat, which is relatively high in iron, and in addition many countries, including the U.S., have mandatory iron fortification of foods. In the U.S., all flour, corn meal, rice, and farina must by law be fortified with iron.

So don't think you'll avoid iron by eating less red meat. It will help, but if you substitute iron-fortified foods, then it may be for naught.

Not all of the iron in food is absorbed into the body, however, and the fraction of iron absorbed can vary tremendously.

That means that you can manipulate your food and drink to decrease the amount of iron that you absorb.

A short list of food and drink that can inhibit iron absorption includes:

- eggs

- dairy products
- grains and vegetables
- foods high in phytates, such as walnuts, almonds, and legumes (beans, peas, lentils)
- tea and coffee
- chocolate
- red wine
- olive oil

Consuming eggs and dairy products with meals can hinder iron absorption as much as 50%. In dairy products, calcium competes for iron absorption, inhibiting it. Eggs contain a substance that tightly binds iron, the same substance that protects eggs from bacterial invasion by denying iron to the invaders.

Tea and coffee greatly lower the amount of iron that's absorbed from a meal. Drinking a cup of coffee with a meal lowers iron absorption by as much as 80%.[142] Curiously, for whatever reason, instant coffee is more potent in this regard than drip coffee. No effect is seen when coffee is drunk before a meal; to inhibit iron, the coffee or tea must be drunk with or shortly after a meal.

Tea (black or green) appears to be the best iron inhibitor.[143] Black tea inhibits iron absorption by up to 94% when drunk with a meal. Adding milk or cream to the tea does not affect its iron-inhibiting ability.

Cocoa or chocolate, red wine, and herb teas also inhibit iron, although to a lesser extent, perhaps two thirds of the degree that coffee or tea do.

The active ingredients that inhibit absorption are polyphenols, the same compounds that provide other health benefits.

Since coffee, tea, and chocolate are all associated with better health, inhibition of iron absorption provides a clear mechanism as to why.

> In the Zutphen Elderly Study, of men in the Netherlands, those men in the highest tertile (upper third) of cocoa intake had about *half* the risk of cardiovascular and all-cause mortality as those in the lowest third. In a study published in the New England Journal of Medicine, consumption of two or more cups of coffee daily was associated with a 10 to 15% lower death rate.

Coffee with breakfast, tea with lunch, and red wine with dinner would be a good strategy for lowering iron intake. An enjoyable one, too!

Note that almost all of these inhibitors of iron absorption work to inhibit non-heme iron, which is the type found in plants. Heme iron, which is found in meat, is much more readily absorbed and less easily inhibited. Dairy products appear to be the only food items that substantially inhibit the absorption of heme iron. Thus, eating cheese with a meat meal will hinder iron absorption from meat.

Food and drink that *increase* iron absorption

Some dietary components increase the absorption of iron. Alcohol can increase iron absorption of a meal by 25% compared to no alcohol with the meal. Many alcoholics eventually develop iron overload because of this. Red wine doesn't have this effect, as the polyphenols in it bind to iron. But beer, white wine, and spirits will all increase iron absorption if drunk with a meal.

Vitamin C strongly increases iron absorption. It should not be taken with meals if you want to decrease iron. Likewise, drinks containing it, such as orange juice, do the same. Any acidic drink will also, such as cranberry juice or tomato juice.

Sugar and high-fructose corn syrup strongly increase hormones that in turn increase iron absorption. Soda and other sweet drinks appear to be a good way to get to iron overload.

Breakfast cereals are often iron-fortified, so avoid these for iron lowering. They're even banned in Denmark, which prohibits iron-fortification.

Cooking in a cast-iron skillet adds a small amount of iron to food, perhaps 1 mg or so, especially if the foods are acidic. Cast-iron skillets should be avoided if lowering iron.

Many foods are high in iron but low in absorption. For instance, people deficient in iron are often advised to eat spinach, but other components in spinach hinder iron absorption, so if you're trying to lower iron, I wouldn't worry too much about spinach.

This brings us to a diet that's very good at lowering iron, the Mediterranean diet.

The Mediterranean Diet

The diet of the various peoples around the Mediterranean Sea is associated with better health: less heart disease, cancer, and diabetes.

While food varies a lot depending on the exact location, the Mediterranean diet has been characterized as one that's high in fruit and vegetable intake, fish consumption, the use of olive oil, the drinking of red wine, and with a relatively low amount of red meat. In countries that practice Orthodox Christianity, fasting during many times in the year is also involved.

Dumping Iron

Much of the health benefit of the Mediterranean diet may be due to lower iron consumption and inhibition of iron absorption, resulting in lower body iron.[144]

The Mediterranean diet can decrease fatty liver and increase insulin sensitivity, and lower body iron stores may be involved, since there's good evidence of a link between body iron and both fatty liver and insulin resistance.

Elderly men in Crete, average age 84, who ate a Mediterranean diet had ferritin (iron) levels about half the size – 70 – of men the same age who lived in the Netherlands – at 132. That's enough to make a big difference in health, and it does.

Men in the Netherlands have *four times the rate of death from heart disease* as the men in Crete. These differences cannot be explained by cholesterol, blood pressure, or physical activity, since the differences in these measures between men in the two countries are small.

In the study, the men in Crete had only about one third the incidence of cancer as the men in the Netherlands.[145]

The constituents of the Mediterranean diet inhibit iron absorption. Olive oil, for instance, and red wine, along with a copious intake of fruits and vegetables, do this. Fish is low in iron, and high-iron red meat is not eaten as much.

It looks like the Mediterranean style of eating may be among the best for keeping body iron stores low.

Note that some other ways of eating, such as the Japanese, with low meat intake and consumption of tea and vegetables, are also healthy and have features that keep iron consumption low.

A recent study done in South Korea, which found that those with high ferritin were more likely to be diabetic, also found that in men and women with normal fasting blood sugar had the lowest ferritin levels. A low-iron diet may help explain it.[146]

The American or Western way of eating, with lots of sugar-laden food and drink, and consumption of plenty of meat along with iron-fortified flour and other grains, can be expected to raise iron stores a lot more. And it does. This could be an important reason for the general ill health of Americans compared with some other societies.

A Low-Iron Diet

Is it actually possible not merely to inhibit iron absorption from food, but to lower body iron stores through diet? Yes, it is possible.

While the body has no regulated means of ridding itself of iron, losses of iron from the body are not zero. Sweating, sloughing of skin and intestinal cells, and minor intestinal bleeding all lead to small losses of iron of about 1 mg a day. (And of course, fertile women lose much larger amounts through the menstrual cycle.)

These small iron losses mean that if iron from food is tightly controlled, iron (ferritin) decreases over time.

Doctor and scientist Francesco Facchini, who has done several trials on lowering iron to prevent and cure disease, put a group of patients with diabetic kidney disease on a low-iron diet, and another group on a standard low-protein diet, which is often used in kidney disease.[147] The low-iron diet also restricted carbohydrates.

Of the patients who were placed on the diet, 20% either died or needed dialysis treatment at the end of four years. Of the patients on the low-protein diet, 39% did.

The low-iron diet cut the rate of death or end-stage renal disease in half.

The low-iron, low-carbohydrate diet looked like this:

- 50% reduction of carbohydrate (from the previous level of intake)
- substitution of iron-rich red meats (beef and pork) with iron-poor white meats (poultry and fish) and with protein-enriched food items known to inhibit iron absorption, e.g., dairy, eggs, and soy
- elimination of all beverages other than tea, milk, water, and red wine. Milk was recommended for breakfast. Tea was "highly recommended". Red wine was not

to exceed 150 ml (about 5 ounces) with lunch and 150 ml with dinner. Outside mealtimes, water was the only approved beverage

- exclusive use of polyphenol-enriched extra-virgin olive oil for both dressing and frying

The diet was not restricted in calories, and even a 50% cut in carbohydrates doesn't make it a true, low-carbohydrate diet in the style of, say, the Atkins diet. Note that total red wine consumption is nearly half a bottle a day. This low-iron diet bears striking similarities to the Mediterranean diet.

By two years into the diet, ferritin dropped from an average of 301 to 36, well into the low normal range, while in the control group, there was no change.

The low-carbohydrate aspect of the diet may have eliminated much of the iron-fortified flour foods, such as bread, and similar items such as breakfast cereal.

Eating low-iron poultry and fish instead of high-iron beef and pork, and eating dairy or eggs with meals, also lowers iron intake.

Especially, the drinking of tea and red wine with meals would substantially inhibit iron absorption. Tea inhibits iron absorption by up to 95%, while red wine inhibits it at about 65%. Note that tea was "highly recommended".

Coffee has nearly the same effect, so if you want to follow a diet like this and prefer coffee to tea, that would work well.

Finally, the exclusive use of olive oil for dressing and cooking would result in a further reduction of iron.

The ferritin level reached by this diet is similar to that seen in lacto-ovo vegetarians, who eat dairy and eggs but not meat. So if you're a meat eater, as most of us are, you can still lower iron levels to safe levels – but you won't be eating many hamburgers or steaks.

If you did nothing but drank tea, coffee, or red wine at meals and lowered your intake of beef and pork, you would likely get much of the iron-lowering benefits of this diet.

To my mind, the one disadvantage with this diet is that it took up to two years to bring ferritin levels down to a low normal level. If I had a ferritin of 300, which was the average in this group, I would want to get it lower more quickly, given what I know about its health benefits. Also keep in mind that many people have a much higher ferritin than 300, so getting it lower via diet will take even longer.

Nevertheless, this diet is a good strategy for lowering iron, especially when used together with other methods, and will work well in keeping it low.

Dose times duration determines iron toxicity

As mentioned, the low-iron diet takes a while to lower body iron stores, up to two years even when followed strictly. This is because natural iron losses, outside of fertile women, are normally quite low. If someone has a high ferritin level, getting it lower quicker is better for health.

That's because the toxicity of iron is a function of the dose of iron – the amount in the body – times the duration – the length of time it's been there.

So the sooner you know your iron level, the faster you can do something about it. While an elderly person with a high iron can improve his or her health by taking measures to lower it, that person would have been better off if it had been discovered earlier.

Iron stores in men start to increase at about the age of 19, and rise to average adult levels by their mid-30s. Iron rises in women starting at about age 50. It would be wise for any man in his 20s, or any woman in her 50s, to know their ferritin levels so that they can begin to take action if necessary.

The iron-lowering interventions described above vary in the speed of lowering iron. Blood donation is the fastest; in theory, given a high rate of donation (once every two months), a donor could lower ferritin by 200 or more points a year. A low-iron diet, on the other hand, could take several years to accomplish the same result. As for iron chelation and inhibition of iron absorption, too many variables are in play to give a satisfactory answer to how long they take to lower iron to a safe level.

It would be a good idea to keep a record of both ferritin levels and the measures taken to lower them. If you undertake a program to lower your iron, you could ask your doctor for standing orders to get your ferritin tested, so that you wouldn't have to see the doctor every time you wanted to do so. By monitoring ferritin as well as the measures taken to lower it, it's possible to keep ferritin in an acceptable range, without going into iron deficiency or iron overload.

Takeaway points

- The normal range and the optimal range of iron are not the same
- The normal range underestimates health risks, which start within the normal range
- Most doctors won't look twice at ferritin values within the normal range, so attaining optimal iron levels

requires some effort on your part

- Blood donation is the surest and quickest way to lower excessive iron

- Natural iron chelators, all of which have health benefits, attach to iron in the body and remove it

- Aspirin dramatically lowers cancer risk, and lowering iron may be the main way it does so.

- Tea, coffee, dairy products, and several other food and drink items can greatly lower the absorption of iron from food

- The Mediterranean diet's health benefits may be due partly or wholly to lowering iron

- A diet low in iron and with added iron blockers like tea and red wine is effective at lowering ferritin, and lowers the death rate in people with kidney disease

8: Conclusion

The accumulation of iron leads to increased aging and worse health, and is involved in causing many diseases, including cancer, heart disease, diabetes, brain disorders, and more.

Taking control of your iron level and ensuring that it doesn't get too high could be one of the most important things you do for your health. It's almost certainly the most important thing that no one ever talks about.

How important is lowering body iron stores compared to other well-known health interventions, like, say, exercise? It's difficult to give a satisfactory answer to that question, but I think that lowering iron could be qualified as "necessary but not sufficient".

If you exercise, maintain a normal body weight, avoid sugar and refined carbohydrates in your diet, get a good night's sleep, and have good health practices in other areas, but you have a high iron level, then I believe that a high iron level may override and negate your good health practices.

If you have poor health practices, are overweight, don't exercise, and eat junk, will having a low iron level save you? No, it will not. It may help a little, but your poor health practices may override your low iron to a great extent.

For optimal health, maintaining low normal body iron stores should be incorporated into a suite of good health practices.

Recognition of the damaging effects of iron is low, even among scientists who study aging and disease, and even among doctors. I hope this book will increase recognition of excess iron as a major source of health risk.

The FDA, the USDA, the WHO, and other government agencies both American and elsewhere will not be coming to the rescue. Except in cases of gross iron overload, such as in hemochromatosis or a history of multiple transfusions, they don't recognize excess iron as a problem. As pointed out several times in this book, pharmaceutical companies have no incentive to investigate this problem.

The most important issue in excess iron is to prevent iron from rising in the first place. For that to happen, there must be a huge increase in awareness of the problem. If there were more awareness, people would be much more skeptical about iron supplements and iron fortification of foods. They would be aware of the health benefits of blood donation and the use of natural phytochemicals such as curcumin or green tea extract.

Legally mandated iron fortification of foods could be slowly poisoning many people. The purported benefit is to a small fraction of the population, those at risk for iron deficiency. Both Sweden (in 1995) and Denmark (in 1987) banned the fortification of foods with iron, mainly because the risks to the majority far outweighed the benefits to the minority. Denmark does not even allow the importation of iron-fortified breakfast cereals on the grounds that they may be harmful.

I wouldn't hold my breath waiting for the end of iron fortification in the U.S. The food lobbyists are too entrenched and there's little recognition of excess iron as a problem. On the contrary, the only recognition of iron as a problem is in the case of iron deficiency, which affects relatively few. The general opinion among both medical professionals and lay people alike is that you just can't get too much iron, and the more the better.

Therefore, to control your iron, you have to take matters into your own hands. Fortunately, this is readily done, although the rather large fraction of the public who are ineligible to donate blood will have to use slower, less efficient methods to lower their iron. Just don't expect to have your doctor bring all of this to your attention because in all likelihood, he or she will not.

To live into your nineties or beyond, with no cancer or heart disease or other major illness, then you must ensure that your body iron stores are not excessive, and preferably within the ranges discussed in this book. Other aspects of health are important, such as exercise, staying lean, and eating a healthy diet, but if you do all those things and don't control your iron, they could end up being exercises in futility.

Appendix: The Men Who Discovered the Iron Connection

The work of a number of scientists and doctors has been important in the discovery and elucidation of the connection between iron and disease. We would know far less about iron and health were it not for their contributions. Following are a few of the most important of these doctors and scientists.

Jerome L. Sullivan, M.D., PhD

Pride of place must go to the late Dr. Jerome Sullivan, a physician and pathologist, who first conceived the iron hypothesis of heart disease. He had been "puzzled" by the fact that men have much higher rates of heart disease than women, and why the rates for women increased after menopause. Until then, and to an extent even now, it was thought that the difference in sex hormones between men and women, and between pre- and post-menopausal women, was the reason.

In 1981, Dr. Sullivan published a seminal paper, "Iron and the sex difference in heart disease risk" in the medical journal *The Lancet*. This paper has been cited by other scientists 759 times as of this writing, and it greatly changed thinking on both iron and heart disease.

Dr. Sullivan went on to write many more scientific papers (86, according to Google Scholar). He lived in Florida and died in 2013.

Francesco Facchini, M.D.

Dr. Francesco Facchini is a doctor now retired from the University of California, San Francisco, and he made the connection between iron and insulin resistance. He has done several studies in which patients or volunteers had their iron lowered, either through phlebotomy or diet.

Dr. Facchini's publications include:

Effect of iron depletion in carbohydrate-intolerant patients with clinical evidence of nonalcoholic fatty liver disease (2002)

Low iron status and enhanced insulin sensitivity in lacto-ovo vegetarians (2001)

A low-iron-available, polyphenol-enriched, carbohydrate-restricted diet to slow progression of diabetic nephropathy (2003)

Effect of iron depletion on cardiovascular risk factors (2002)

Near-iron deficiency-induced remission of gouty arthritis

(2003)

Eugene D. Weinberg, PhD

Dr. Eugene Weinberg is Professor Emeritus of Biology at the University of Indiana. His career was devoted to studying the biological actions of iron and other trace metals, and he's written extensively on the dangers of excessive iron. He is the author of over 140 scientific papers.

Among Dr. Weinberg's publications:

Iron availability and infection (2009)

Iron loading: a risk factor for osteoporosis (2006)

The hazards of iron loading (2010)

The role of iron in cancer (1996)

Leo R. Zacharski, M.D.

Dr. Leo Zacharski is Professor of Medicine, Geisel School of Medicine at Dartmouth College, and heads an iron overload clinic at the Hitchcock Hospital, Lebanon, NH. He's done important work on the toxicity of ambient levels of body iron stores, and has conducted clinical trials of lowering iron.

Among Dr. Zacharski's publications:

Reducing iron stores lowers cancer risk in patients with

peripheral arterial disease (2007)

Reduction of Iron Stores and Cardiovascular Outcomes in Patients with Peripheral Arterial Disease (2007)

Association of age, sex, and race with body iron stores in adults: analysis of NHANES III data (2000)

Getting the iron out: Phlebotomy for Alzheimer's disease? (2009)

Luca Mascitelli, M.D.

Dr. Luca Mascitelli is both a physician and a Lieutenant Colonel in the Italian Army. In the course of my research on iron and health, I came across numerous articles and letters by him on this topic. He has been tireless in drawing attention to the hazards of iron regarding many medical conditions.

Several of his publications were co-authored with the late Dr. Jerome Sullivan.

Among Dr. Mascitelli's publications:

Explaining sex difference in coronary heart disease: is it time to shift from the oestrogen hypothesis to the iron hypothesis? (2011)

Inhibition of Iron Absorption by Coffee and the Reduced Risk of Type 2 Diabetes Mellitus (2007)

Aspirin-associated iron loss as an anticancer mechanism (2010)

Is the Beneficial Antioxidant Effect of Olive Oil Mediated by Interaction of its Phenolic Constituents and Iron? (2010)

The Mediterranean Diet and Body Iron Stores (2014)

Acknowledgments

I would like to thank the following people for their help and support.

Eugene D. Weinberg, PhD, for granting an interview and for writing the foreword to this book.

Lt. Colonel Luca Mascitelli, M.D., for correspondence, supplying me with his (pay-walled) articles, and for writing a recommendation of this book.

Leo Zacharski, M.D., who went way above and beyond my expectations in his help and enthusiasm for this book, and for writing the preface.

Jay Campbell, physique trainer and testosterone therapy advocate extraordinaire, of FabFitOver40.com, for his support.

David Goodman, of TheSurvivalGardener.com, for suggesting the title, designing the cover, and for sharing his book-marketing expertise.

Francesco Facchini, M.D., for correspondence and writing a recommendation for this book.

My readers and Twitter followers, who have been a tremendous source of goodwill and support.

And of course, Michele.

About the Author

P. D. (Dennis) Mangan has a background in microbiology and pharmacology. He lives in California, where he lifts weights in a run-down gym.

Dumping Iron is his sixth book on health and fitness. His other books are (in reverse order)

- [Muscle Up: How Strength Training Beats Obesity, Cancer, and Heart Disease, and Why Everyone Should Do It](#)
- [Stop the Clock: The Optimal Anti-Aging Program](#)
- [Top Ten Reasons We're Fat](#)
- [Best Supplements for Men's Health, Strength, and Virility](#)
- [Smash Chronic Fatigue](#)

All of these are available at Amazon.com.

You can find more of his writing on health, fitness, and anti-aging at his website, **Rogue Health and Fitness**. Subscribe to the site and get a free guide to intermittent fasting.

If you liked this book, please leave a review at the book's Amazon.com web page.

Bibliography

1. Hansen JB1, Tonnesen MF, Madsen AN, et al. Cell Metab. 2012 Oct 3;16(4):449-61. doi: 10.1016/j.cmet.2012.09.001. Epub 2012 Sep 20. Divalent metal transporter 1 regulates iron-mediated ROS and pancreatic cell fate in response to cytokines.
2. Zacharski LR. Ferrotoxic disease: the next great public health challenge. Clin Chem 2014;60:1362-4
3. Ferrotoxic disease: quantitative effects of iron excess on health: www.healtheiron.com Accessed February 12, 2016
4. Schümann K, Ettle T, Szegner B, Elsenhans B, Solomons NW. On risks and benefits of iron supplementation recommendations for iron intake revisited. J Trace Elem Med Biol. 2007;21(3):147-68. Epub 2007 Aug 1.
5. Zacharski LR, Shamayeva G, Chow BK, DePalma RG. Racial health disparities, and variant Red Cell and Iron homeostasis. JHCPU May 2015.
6. Pachón H, Spohrer R, Mei Z, Serdula MK. Evidence of the effectiveness of flour fortification programs on iron status and anemia: a systematic review. Nutr Rev. 2015 Nov;73(11):780-95. doi: 10.1093/nutrit/nuv037. Epub 2015 Oct 2.
7. Fleming DJ, Tucker KL, Jacques PF, et al. Dietary factors associated with the risk of high iron stores in the elderly Framingham Heart Study cohort. Am J Clin Nutr 2002;76:1375-84.
8. Cook, Christopher I., and Byung Pal Yu. "Iron accumulation in aging: modulation by dietary restriction." Mechanisms of Ageing and Development 102.1 (1998): 1-13.
9. Reverter-Branchat, Gemma, et al. "Oxidative damage to specific proteins in replicative and chronological-aged Saccharomyces cerevisiae common targets and prevention by calorie restriction." Journal of Biological Chemistry 279.30 (2004): 31983-31989.

10   Mori, Nobuko, and Kimiko Hirayama. "Long-term consumption of a methionine-supplemented diet increases iron and lipid peroxide levels in rat liver." The Journal of Nutrition 130.9 (2000): 2349-2355.
11   Massie, Harold R., Valerie R. Aiello, and Trevor R. Williams. "Inhibition of iron absorption prolongs the life span of Drosophila." Mechanisms of Ageing and Development 67.3 (1993): 227-237.
12   Schiavi, Alfonso, et al. "Iron-starvation-induced mitophagy mediates lifespan extension upon mitochondrial stress in C. elegans." Current Biology 25.14 (2015): 1810-1822.   Klang, Ida M., et al. "Iron promotes protein insolubility and aging in C. elegans." Aging (Albany NY) 6.11 (2014): 975.

13   Hatcher, Heather C., et al. "Synthetic and natural iron chelators: therapeutic potential and clinical use." Future Medicinal Chemistry 1.9 (2009): 1643-1670.
14   Forte, Giovanni, et al. "Metals in plasma of nonagenarians and centenarians living in a key area of longevity." Experimental Gerontology 60 (2014): 197-206.
15   Zacharski, Leo R., et al. "Association of age, sex, and race with body iron stores in adults: analysis of NHANES III data." American Heart Journal 140.1 (2000): 98-104.
16   Sullivan, Jerome L. "Are menstruating women protected from heart disease because of, or in spite of, estrogen? Relevance to the iron hypothesis."American Heart Journal 145.2 (2003): 190-194.
17   Salonen, Jukka T., et al. "Donation of blood is associated with reduced risk of myocardial infarction The Kuopio Ischaemic Heart Disease Risk Factor Study." American Journal of Epidemiology 148.5 (1998): 445-451.
18   Meyers, David G., et al. "Possible association of a reduction in cardiovascular events with blood donation." Heart 78.2 (1997): 188-193.
19   Meyers, David G., Kelly C. Jensen, and Jay E. Menitove. "A historical cohort study of the effect of lowering body iron through blood donation on incident cardiac events." Transfusion 42.9 (2002): 1135-1139.
20   Ullum, Henrik, et al. "Blood donation and blood donor mortality after adjustment for a healthy donor effect." Transfusion 55.10 (2015): 2479-2485.
21   Ellervik, Christina, et al. "Total and cause-specific mortality by moderately and markedly increased ferritin concentrations: general population study and metaanalysis." Clinical Chemistry 60.11 (2014): 1419-1428.

22   Kurz, Tino, Alexei Terman, and Ulf T. Brunk. "Autophagy, ageing and apoptosis: the role of oxidative stress and lysosomal iron." Archives of Biochemistry and Biophysics 462.2 (2007): 220-230.
23   Wiley, Christopher D., et al. "Mitochondrial Dysfunction Induces Senescence with a Distinct Secretory Phenotype." Cell Metabolism (2015).
24   Walter, Patrick B., et al. "Iron deficiency and iron excess damage mitochondria and mitochondrial DNA in rats." Proceedings of the National Academy of Sciences 99.4 (2002): 2264-2269.
25   Troutt, Jason S., et al. "Circulating human hepcidin-25 concentrations display a diurnal rhythm, increase with prolonged fasting, and are reduced by growth hormone administration." Clinical Chemistry 58.8 (2012): 1225-1232.
26   Shang, Chaowei, Hongyu Zhou, and Shile Huang. "Iron chelation inhibits mTOR activity in cancer cells." Cancer Research 74.19 Supplement (2014): 2789-2789.
27   Roecker, L., et al. "Iron-regulatory protein hepcidin is increased in female athletes after a marathon." European Journal of Applied Physiology 95.5-6 (2005): 569-571.
28   Peeling, Peter, et al. "Iron status and the acute post-exercise hepcidin response in athletes." PloS One 9.3 (2014): e93002.
29   De Valk, B., and J. J. M. Marx. "Iron, atherosclerosis, and ischemic heart disease." Archives of Internal Medicine 159.14 (1999): 1542-1548. [Much of the chapter on heart disease is based on this paper.]
30   Sullivan, Jerome L. "The iron paradigm of ischemic heart disease." American Heart Journal 117.5 (1989): 1177-1188.
31   Salonen, Jukka T., et al. "High stored iron levels are associated with excess risk of myocardial infarction in eastern Finnish men." Circulation 86.3 (1992): 803-811.
32   Sullivan, Jerome L. "Are menstruating women protected from heart disease because of, or in spite of, estrogen? Relevance to the iron hypothesis."American Heart Journal 145.2 (2003): 190-194.
33   Mascitelli, L., and M. R. Goldstein. "Might the beneficial effects of statin drugs be related to their action on iron metabolism?." QJM 105.12 (2012): 1225-1229.
34   Zacharski, Leo R., et al. "The statin–iron nexus: anti-inflammatory intervention for arterial disease prevention." American Journal of Public Health103.4 (2013): e105-e112.
35   Lauffer, R. B. "Iron stores and the international variation in mortality from coronary artery disease." Medical Hypotheses 35.2 (1991): 96-102.
36   https://www.hsph.harvard.edu/news/features/edgren-cancer-sex-differences/

37 Mascitelli, Luca, and Mark R. Goldstein. "Explaining sex difference in cancer risk: Might it be related to excess iron?." International Journal of Cancer133.9 (2013): 2261-2262.
38 Zacharski, Leo R., et al. "Decreased cancer risk after iron reduction in patients with peripheral arterial disease: results from a randomized trial."Journal of the National Cancer Institute 100.14 (2008): 996-1002.
39 Knekt, Paul, et al. "Body iron stores and risk of cancer." International Journal of Cancer 56.3 (1994): 379-382.
40 Stevens, Richard G., R. Palmer Beasley, and Baruch S. Blumberg. "Iron-binding proteins and risk of cancer in Taiwan." Journal of the National Cancer Institute 76.4 (1986): 605-610.
41 Wu, Tiejian, et al. "Serum iron, copper and zinc concentrations and risk of cancer mortality in US adults." Annals of epidemiology 14.3 (2004): 195-201.
42 Raina, Komal, et al. "Inositol hexaphosphate inhibits tumor growth, vascularity, and metabolism in TRAMP mice: a multiparametric magnetic resonance study." Cancer Prevention Research 6.1 (2013): 40-50.
43 Yuan, Jun, David B. Lovejoy, and Des R. Richardson. "Novel di-2-pyridyl–derived iron chelators with marked and selective antitumor activity: in vitro and in vivo assessment." Blood 104.5 (2004): 1450-1458.
44 Torti, Suzy V., and Frank M. Torti. "Iron and cancer: more ore to be mined."Nature Reviews Cancer 13.5 (2013): 342-355.
45 Mascitelli, Luca, Francesca Pezzetta, and Jerome L. Sullivan. "Aspirin-associated iron loss as an anticancer mechanism." Medical hypotheses 74.1 (2010): 78-80.
46 Rothwell, Peter M., et al. "Effect of daily aspirin on risk of cancer metastasis: a study of incident cancers during randomised controlled trials."The Lancet 379.9826 (2012): 1591-1601.
47 Stellman, Steven D., et al. "Smoking and lung cancer risk in American and Japanese men: an international case-control study." Cancer Epidemiology Biomarkers & Prevention 10.11 (2001): 1193-1199.
48 McCormack, Valerie A., et al. "Aspirin and NSAID use and lung cancer risk: a pooled analysis in the International Lung Cancer Consortium (ILCCO)."Cancer Causes & Control 22.12 (2011): 1709-1720.
49 Chanvorachote, Pithi, and Sudjit Luanpitpong. "Iron Induces Cancer Stem Cells and Aggressive Phenotypes in Human Lung Cancer Cells." American Journal of Physiology-Cell Physiology (2016): ajpcell-00322.
50 Ninomiya, Takayuki, et al. "Iron control is a novel therapeutic target of cancer stem cells." Cancer Research 75.15 Supplement (2015): 4243-4243.

51 Toyokuni, Shinya. "Role of iron in carcinogenesis: cancer as a ferrotoxic disease." Cancer science 100.1 (2009): 9-16.
52 Weinberg, E. D. "Tobacco smoke iron: an initiator/promoter of multiple diseases." Biometals 22.2 (2009): 207-210.
53 Weinberg, E. D. "The role of iron in cancer." Eur J Cancer Prev 5.1 (1996): 19-36.
54 Connor, J. R., et al. "A histochemical study of iron, transferrin, and ferritin in Alzheimer's diseased brains." Journal of neuroscience research 31.1 (1992): 75-83.
55 Raven, E. P., et al. "Increased iron levels and decreased tissue integrity in hippocampus of Alzheimer's disease detected in vivo with magnetic resonance imaging." Journal of Alzheimer's disease: JAD 37.1 (2013): 127.
56 Butterfield, D. Allan, Fabio Di Domenico, and Eugenio Barone. "Elevated risk of type 2 diabetes for development of Alzheimer disease: a key role for oxidative stress in brain." Biochimica et Biophysica Acta (BBA)-Molecular Basis of Disease 1842.9 (2014): 1693-1706.
57 Mandel, Silvia, et al. "Iron dysregulation in Alzheimer's disease: multimodal brain permeable iron chelating drugs, possessing neuroprotective-neurorescue and amyloid precursor protein-processing regulatory activities as therapeutic agents." *Progress in neurobiology* 82.6 (2007): 348-360.
58 Ayton, Scott, et al. "Ferritin levels in the cerebrospinal fluid predict Alzheimer/'s disease outcomes and are regulated by APOE." Nature communications 6 (2015).
59 Bartzokis, George, et al. "Prevalent iron metabolism gene variants associated with increased brain ferritin iron in healthy older men." *Journal of Alzheimer's Disease* 20.1 (2010): 333-341.
60 Pisa, Diana, et al. "Different Brain Regions are Infected with Fungi in Alzheimer's Disease." Scientific reports 5 (2015).
61 Weinreb, Orly, et al. "Targeting dysregulation of brain iron homeostasis in Parkinson's disease by iron chelators." Free Radical Biology and Medicine62 (2013): 52-64.
62 de Lima, Maria Noemia Martins, et al. "Selegiline protects against recognition memory impairment induced by neonatal iron treatment."Experimental Neurology 196.1 (2005): 177-183.
63 Bartzokis, George, et al. "Brain ferritin iron may influence age-and gender-related risks of neurodegeneration." Neurobiology of Aging 28.3 (2007): 414-423.
64 Smith, Mark A., et al. "Increased iron and free radical generation in preclinical Alzheimer disease and mild cognitive impairment." Journal of Alzheimer's disease: JAD 19.1 (2010): 363.

65 Dwyer, Barney E., et al. "Getting the iron out: Phlebotomy for Alzheimer's disease?." Medical Hypotheses 72.5 (2009): 504-509.

66 Mandel, Silvia, et al. "Green tea catechins as brain-permeable, natural iron chelators-antioxidants for the treatment of neurodegenerative disorders."Molecular nutrition & food research 50.2 (2006): 229-234.

67 Xu, Qi, Anumantha G. Kanthasamy, and Manju B. Reddy. "Neuroprotective effect of the natural iron chelator, phytic acid in a cell culture model of Parkinson's disease." Toxicology 245.1 (2008): 101-108.

68 Iwasaki, Tomoyuki, et al. "Serum ferritin is associated with visceral fat area and subcutaneous fat area." Diabetes Care 28.10 (2005): 2486-2491.

69 Gillum, R. F. "Association of serum ferritin and indices of body fat distribution and obesity in Mexican American men—the Third National Health and Nutrition Examination Survey." International Journal of Obesity & Related Metabolic Disorders 25.5 (2001).

70 Ukkola, Olavi, and Merja Santaniemi. "Adiponectin: a link between excess adiposity and associated comorbidities?." Journal of Molecular Medicine80.11 (2002): 696-702.

71 Gabrielsen, J. Scott, et al. "Adipocyte iron regulates adiponectin and insulin sensitivity." The Journal of clinical investigation 122.10 (2012): 3529.

72 Facchini, Francesco S., Nancy W. Hua, and Riccardo A. Stoohs. "Effect of iron depletion in carbohydrate-intolerant patients with clinical evidence of nonalcoholic fatty liver disease." Gastroenterology 122.4 (2002): 931-939.

73 Bailey, Regan L., et al. "Dietary supplement use in the United States, 2003-2006." The Journal of nutrition (2010): jn-110.

74 Topaloglu, A. Kemal, et al. "Lack of association between plasma leptin levels and appetite in children with iron deficiency." Nutrition 17.7 (2001): 657-659.

75 Gao, Yan, et al. "Adipocyte iron regulates leptin and food intake." The Journal of Clinical Investigation 125.9 (2015): 3681-3691.

76 http://www.cnpp.usda.gov/sites/default/files/nutrient_content_of_the_us_food_supply/FoodSupply1909-2000.pdf

77 Christides, Tatiana, and Paul Sharp. "Sugars increase non-heme iron bioavailability in human epithelial intestinal and liver cells." PloS one 8.12 (2013): e83031.

78 Weinberg, Eugene D. "Iron availability and infection." Biochimica et Biophysica Acta (BBA)-General Subjects 1790.7 (2009): 600-605.

79 Weinberg, Eugene D. "Iron loading and disease surveillance." Emerging infectious diseases 5.3 (1999): 346.

[80] Azar, Sima Abedi, and Mohammad Reza Jafari Nakhjavani. "The effect of intravenous iron on bacterial infection in hemodialysis patients." *Life Science Journal* 12.3s (2015).
[81] Bullen, John, et al. "Sepsis: the critical role of iron." Microbes and infection2.4 (2000): 409-415.
[82] Zager, Richard A., Ali CM Johnson, and Sherry Y. Hanson. "Parenteral iron therapy exacerbates experimental sepsis Rapid Communication." Kidney international 65.6 (2004): 2108-2112.
[83] Islam, Sufia, et al. "Anti-inflammatory and anti-bacterial effects of iron chelation in experimental sepsis." Journal of Surgical Research 200.1 (2016): 266-273.
[84] Osthoff, Michael, et al. "Low-Dose Acetylsalicylic Acid Treatment and Impact on Short-Term Mortality in Staphylococcus aureus Bloodstream Infection: A Propensity Score-Matched Cohort Study." Critical care medicine(2016).
[85] Singh, Ajay Vikram, and Paolo Zamboni. "Anomalous venous blood flow and iron deposition in multiple sclerosis." Journal of Cerebral Blood Flow & Metabolism 29.12 (2009): 1867-1878.
[86] http://yourmedicalguide.info/italian-doctor-may-have-found-surprisingly-simple-cure-for-multiple-sclerosis/
[87] Facchini, Francesco S. "Near-iron deficiency-induced remission of gouty arthritis." Rheumatology 42.12 (2003): 1550-1555.
[88] Weinberg, E. D. "Tobacco smoke iron: an initiator/promoter of multiple diseases." Biometals 22.2 (2009): 207-210.
[89] Cloonan, Suzanne M., et al. "Mitochondrial iron chelation ameliorates cigarette smoke-induced bronchitis and emphysema in mice." Nature medicine (2016).
[90] Reid, David William, Greg J. Anderson, and Iain L. Lamont. "Role of lung iron in determining the bacterial and host struggle in cystic fibrosis." American Journal of Physiology-Lung Cellular and Molecular Physiology 297.5 (2009): L795-L802.
[91] Bugianesi, Elisabetta, et al. "Relative contribution of iron burden, HFE mutations, and insulin resistance to fibrosis in nonalcoholic fatty liver."Hepatology 39.1 (2004): 179-187.
[92] Valenti, Luca, et al. "A randomized trial of iron depletion in patients with nonalcoholic fatty liver disease and hyperferritinemia." World journal of gastroenterology: WJG 20.11 (2014): 3002.
[93] Garg, R., Z. Goodman, and Z. Younossi. "Commentary: phlebotomy in non-alcoholic fatty liver disease." Alimentary Pharmacology & Therapeutics 37.11 (2013): 1112-1112.
[94] https://www.ncbi.nlm.nih.gov/pubmed/11808931

95 Yano, Motoyoshi, et al. "Long term effects of phlebotomy on biochemical and histological parameters of chronic hepatitis C." The American Journal of Gastroenterology 97.1 (2002): 133-137.
96 Kato, Junji, et al. "Long-term phlebotomy with low-iron diet therapy lowers risk of development of hepatocellular carcinoma from chronic hepatitis C."Journal of Gastroenterology 42.10 (2007): 830-836.
97 Kohgo, Yutaka, et al. "Iron accumulation in alcoholic liver diseases."Alcoholism: Clinical and Experimental Research 29.s2 (2005): 189S-193S.
98 Irving, Michael G., June W. Halliday, and Lawrie W. Powell. "Association between alcoholism and increased hepatic iron stores." Alcoholism: Clinical and Experimental Research 12.1 (1988): 7-13.
99 Ritter, Cristiane, et al. "Protective effect of N-acetylcysteine and deferoxamine on carbon tetrachloride-induced acute hepatic failure in rats."Critical Care Medicine 32.10 (2004): 2079-2083.
100 Marzetti, Emanuele, et al. "Sarcopenia of aging: underlying cellular mechanisms and protection by calorie restriction." Biofactors 35.1 (2009): 28-35.
101 Xu, Jinze, et al. "Iron accumulation with age, oxidative stress and functional decline." PLoS One 3.8 (2008): e2865-e2865.
102 Kim, Tae Ho, Hee-Jin Hwang, and Sang-Hwan Kim. "Relationship between serum ferritin levels and sarcopenia in Korean females aged 60 years and older using the fourth Korea National Health and Nutrition Examination Survey (KNHANES IV-2, 3), 2008-2009." PloS one 9.2 (2014).
103 Weinberg, Eugene D. "Iron loading: a risk factor for osteoporosis." Biometals19.6 (2006): 633-635.
104 Jian, Jinlong, Edward Pelle, and Xi Huang. "Iron and menopause: does increased iron affect the health of postmenopausal women?." Antioxidants & redox signaling 11.12 (2009): 2939-2943.
105 Liu, Gang, et al. "Therapeutic effects of an oral chelator targeting skeletal tissue damage in experimental postmenopausal osteoporosis in rats."Hemoglobin 32.1-2 (2008): 181-190.
106 Dunaief, Joshua L. "Iron induced oxidative damage as a potential factor in age-related macular degeneration: the Cogan Lecture." Investigative ophthalmology & visual science 47.11 (2006): 4660-4664.
107 Pelle, Edward, et al. "Menopause increases the iron storage protein ferritin in skin." Journal of cosmetic science 64.3 (2012): 175-179.

108 Pourzand, Charareh, et al. "Ultraviolet A radiation induces immediate release of iron in human primary skin fibroblasts: the role of ferritin." Proceedings of the National Academy of Sciences 96.12 (1999): 6751-6756.

109 Bissett, Donald L., Ranjit Chatterjee, and Daniel P. Hannon. "Chronic ultraviolet radiation-induced increase in skin iron and the photoprotective effect of topically applied iron chelators 1,*." Photochemistry and Photobiology 54.2 (1991): 215-223.

110 Stegeman, Bernardine H., et al. "Different combined oral contraceptives and the risk of venous thrombosis: systematic review and network meta-analysis." Bmj 347 (2013): f5298.

111 Beaber, Elisabeth F., et al. "Oral contraceptives and breast cancer risk overall and by molecular subtype among young women." Cancer Epidemiology Biomarkers & Prevention 23.5 (2014): 755-764.

112 Larsson, Gerd, et al. "The influence of a low-dose combined oral contraceptive on menstrual blood loss and iron status." Contraception 46.4 (1992): 327-334.

113 Milman, N., M. Kirchhoff, and T. Jørgensen. "Iron status markers, serum ferritin and hemoglobin in 1359 Danish women in relation to menstruation, hormonal contraception, parity, and postmenopausal hormone treatment."Annals of Hematology 65.2 (1992): 96-102.

114 Weinberg, E. D. "First trimester curtailment of iron absorption: Innate suppression of a teratogen?." Medical hypotheses 74.2 (2010): 246-247.

115 Naieni, Farahnaz Fatemi, et al. "Serum iron, zinc, and copper concentration in premature graying of hair." *Biological trace element research* 146.1 (2012): 30-34.

116 Ganz, Tomas, and Elizabeta Nemeth. "Hepcidin and iron homeostasis."Biochimica et Biophysica Acta (BBA)-Molecular Cell Research 1823.9 (2012): 1434-1443.

117 http://www.labdiet.com/cs/groups/lolweb/@labdiet/documents/web_content/mdrf/mdi4/~edisp/ducm04_028438.pdf

118 Naigamwalla, Dinaz Z., Jinelle A. Webb, and Urs Giger. "Iron deficiency anemia." Can Vet J 53.3 (2012): 250-256.

119 http://www.labdiet.com/cs/groups/lolweb/@labdiet/documents/web_content/mdrf/mdi4/~edisp/ducm04_028202.pdf

120 http://www.aafco.org/Portals/0/SiteContent/Regulatory/Committees/Pet-Food/Reports/Pet_Food_Report_2013_Midyear-Proposed_Revisions_to_AAFCO_Nutrient_Profiles.pdf

121 https://en.wikipedia.org/wiki/Creme_Puff_(cat)
122 Ware, William R. "The Risk of Too Much Iron: Normal Serum Ferritin Levels May Represent Significant Health Issues." Journal of Orthomolecular Medicine 28.4 (2013).
123 Jung, Chang Hee, et al. "Elevated serum ferritin level is associated with the incident type 2 diabetes in healthy Korean men: a 4 year longitudinal study."PloS One 8.9 (2013): e75250.
124 Zhao, Zhuoxian, et al. "Body iron stores and heme-iron intake in relation to risk of type 2 diabetes: a systematic review and meta-analysis." PloS one7.7 (2012): e41641.
125 Ford, Earl S., and Mary E. Cogswell. "Diabetes and serum ferritin concentration among US adults." Diabetes Care 22.12 (1999): 1978-1983.
126 Grobbee, Diederick E., et al. "Serum ferritin is a risk factor for stroke in postmenopausal women." Stroke 36.8 (2005): 1637-1641.
127 Zheng, Haoyi, et al. "Iron stores and vascular function in voluntary blood donors." Arteriosclerosis, thrombosis, and vascular biology 25.8 (2005): 1577-1583.
128 Zacharski, Leo R., et al. "Decreased cancer risk after iron reduction in patients with peripheral arterial disease: results from a randomized trial."Journal of the National Cancer Institute 100.14 (2008): 996-1002.
129 Facchini, Francesco S., Nancy W. Hua, and Riccardo A. Stoohs. "Effect of iron depletion in carbohydrate-intolerant patients with clinical evidence of nonalcoholic fatty liver disease." Gastroenterology 122.4 (2002): 931-939.
130 Ware, William R. "The Risk of Too Much Iron: Normal Serum Ferritin Levels May Represent Significant Health Issues." Journal of Orthomolecular Medicine 28.4 (2013).
[131] Finch, Clement A., et al. "Effect of blood donation on iron stores as evaluated by serum ferritin." *Blood* 50.3 (1977): 441-447.
132 http://usatoday30.usatoday.com/news/nation/2011-08-06-blood-donation-record_n.htm
133 Youdim, Kuresh A., et al. "Flavonoid permeability across an in situ model of the blood–brain barrier." Free Radical Biology and Medicine 36.5 (2004): 592-604.
134 Jiao, Yan, et al. "Iron chelation in the biological activity of curcumin." Free Radical Biology and Medicine 40.7 (2006): 1152-1160.
135 Xu, Qi, Anumantha G. Kanthasamy, and Manju B. Reddy. "Neuroprotective effect of the natural iron chelator, phytic acid in a cell culture model of Parkinson's disease." Toxicology 245.1 (2008): 101-108.

136 Reznichenko, L., et al. "Reduction of iron-regulated amyloid precursor protein and β-amyloid peptide by (–)-epigallocatechin-3-gallate in cell cultures: implications for iron chelation in Alzheimer's disease." Journal of neurochemistry 97.2 (2006): 527-536.

137 Mollet IG, Patel D, Govani FS, Giess A, Paschalaki K, Periyasamy M, et al. (2016) Low Dose Iron Treatments Induce a DNA Damage Response in Human Endothelial Cells within Minutes. PLoS ONE 11(2): e0147990. doi:10.1371/journal.pone.0147990

138 Rothwell, Peter M., et al. "Effect of daily aspirin on long-term risk of death due to cancer: analysis of individual patient data from randomised trials."The Lancet 377.9759 (2011): 31-41.

139 Fleming, Diana J., et al. "Aspirin intake and the use of serum ferritin as a measure of iron status." The American journal of clinical nutrition 74.2 (2001): 219-226.

140 De Berardis G, Lucisano G, D'Ettorre A, et al. Association of Aspirin Use With Major Bleeding in Patients With and Without Diabetes. JAMA. 2012;307(21):2286-2294. doi:10.1001/jama.2012.5034.

141 http://www.nytimes.com/2012/03/21/health/research/studies-link-aspirin-daily-use-to-reduced-cancer-risk.html?src=me&ref=general

142 Morck, Timothy A., S. R. Lynch, and J. D. Cook. "Inhibition of food iron absorption by coffee." The American journal of clinical nutrition 37.3 (1983): 416-420.

143 Hurrell, Richard F., Manju Reddy, and James D. Cook. "Inhibition of non-haem iron absorption in man by polyphenolic-containing beverages." British Journal of Nutrition 81 (1999): 289-295.

144 Mascitelli, Luca, and Mark R. Goldstein. "Might some of the beneficial effects of the Mediterranean diet on non-alcoholic fatty liver disease be mediated by reduced iron stores?." Journal of hepatology 59.3 (2013): 639.

145 Buijsse, Brian, et al. "Oxidative stress, and iron and antioxidant status in elderly men: differences between the Mediterranean south (Crete) and northern Europe (Zutphen)." European Journal of Cardiovascular Prevention & Rehabilitation 14.4 (2007): 495-500.

146 Kim, Chul-Hee, et al. "Association of elevated serum ferritin concentration with insulin resistance and impaired glucose metabolism in Korean men and women." Metabolism 60.3 (2011): 414-420.

147 Facchini, Francesco S., and Kami L. Saylor. "A low-iron-available, polyphenol-enriched, carbohydrate-restricted diet to slow progression of diabetic nephropathy." *Diabetes* 52.5 (2003): 1204-1209.

Made in the USA
Middletown, DE
25 September 2017